DATE DUE

GAYLORD   PRINTED IN U.S.A.

THE SCHWARZBEIN PRINCIPLE COOKBOOK

Diana Schwarzbein, M.D.
Nancy Deville
and Evelyn Jacob Jaffe

Health Communications, Inc.
Deerfield Beach, Florida

www.hci-online.com

Library of Congress Cataloging-in-Publication Data

Schwarzbein, Diana
    The Schwarzbein principle cookbook / Diana Schwarzbein, Nancy Deville and Evelyn Jacob Jaffe.   641.5638
        p.   cm.   SCH
                                                         10.06
    ISBN 1-55874-681-1
    1. Low-carbohydrate diet recipes.   2. Sugar-free diet recipes.   I. Deville, Nancy.   II. Jaffe, Evelyn Jacob.   III. Title.
RM237.73.S35 1999   99-26054
641.5'638—dc21   CIP

©1999 Diana Schwarzbein, M.D., Nancy Deville and Evelyn Jacob Jaffe

ISBN 1-55874-681-1

Publisher: Health Communications, Inc.
        3201 S.W. 15th Street
        Deerfield Beach, FL 33442-8190

Cover design by Lisa Camp
Author photos by Alice Williams

For my mami,
Martha Schwarzbein, who sat with me
for many hours when I was a child,
trying to get me to eat!

—DIANA SCHWARZBEIN, M.D.

For Emma and Charlotte
for their boundless joy and love.

—NANCY DEVILLE

For my mom, Ghislaine Jacob,
my inspiration, and to my dad, "Papa O. J."
for all your encouragement
and love.

—EVELYN JACOB JAFFE

Contents

Acknowledgments

This cookbook is the direct result of a deluge of requests by readers of *The Schwarzbein Principle*. Many, many thanks to our enthusiastic supporters.

We are indebted to a number of people who worked on this project. We are grateful to those who contributed recipes and ideas. We thank Adele Staal, Sheridan Eldridge and all the volunteers from Project Food Chain for experimenting with recipes and giving feedback.

Orien Armstrong, was, as always, a pleasure to work with. David Stanley and Harold "Wardie" Ward gave much-needed computer support. A special thanks to Kelli Tatlock who has been an invaluable assistant during the writing of this book—and for always being cheerful.

From Diana Schwarzbein, M.D., thank you to all my patients for sticking to the program without the benefit of recipes.

From Nancy, sincere thanks to Pat Frederick for her superb editorial skills, attention, support and endurance in the face of unending details—and for being a pleasure to work with. Thanks to Joy Morrison, Reneé Perez and Jillian Jacobs at The Owner Managed Business Institute for clerical support.

From Evelyn, thanks to Joss and Bowie for being such fans of Momma's cooking.

The Schwarzbein Principle Cookbooks would not have been

published if not for Russell Bishop who introduced us to Jack Canfield who, in turn, gave our manuscripts to Peter Vegso at Health Communications, Inc. We are grateful to Peter for believing in our project, and for his infectious enthusiasm. Many thanks to our agent, Barbara Neighbors Deal, for handling the details that went into making our publishing deal.

Peter's staff at HCI made the final editorial process so painless, we actually enjoyed it. We give special acknowledgment to: Christine Belleris, editorial codirector, and Allison Janse, associate editor, who were there with us through thick and thin; Kim Weiss and Maria Konicki in PR; Lisa Camp for the cover design; Erica Orloff for an excellent job copyediting; Lawna Oldfield for the inside book design; Susan Olason for the index; and Teri Peluso, executive assistant, for all of their expertise, support and hard work in getting the book to press.

We also thank Lisa Ekus and Merrilyn Lewis at Lisa Ekus Public Relations for their wonderful efforts on our behalf.

But most of all we are grateful to our husbands, Larry Mousouris, John Davis and Arno Jaffe for their love, patience, understanding and *appetites.*

Introduction

Americans are in constant pursuit of good health. We are deluged with information on how to improve eating and lifestyle habits. We look to "healthier" cultures for the answers. The French, rural Chinese, Inuits, Africans and Tibetans have all been examined in an attempt to understand why they do not suffer the same high rate of chronic degenerative diseases as we do in this country.

The so-called "French paradox" implies that the lower rate of heart disease in the French population, despite their high fat intake, can be attributed to the fact that they drink wine. That must mean drinking a lot of wine is good for you. But the Inuits eat a *high*-fat diet. It must be the fish oils. We need to eat more fish. Africans eat wild game, which is high in saturated fats. But of course they exercise more than we do. We must exercise more. What about the Tibetans, who drink yak-butter tea all day long. Could it be the altitude?

All of these conclusions seem plausible—especially if you still believe that eating a low-fat diet is healthy. But consider the common denominator in these four cultures: The French, Inuits, Africans and Tibetans all eat a diet of "real" foods—foods that they could, in theory, pick, gather, milk, hunt or fish. But equally important: *They eat foods that are rich in good fats.* In other words, these cultures have remained the healthiest in the world because they have *not* gone on low-fat diets.

If you have read *The Schwarzbein Principle* you know why eating a low-fat diet, high in carbohydrates and stimulants, is the major factor in the rise in chronic degenerative diseases in our country.

What You Will Learn When You Read *The Schwarzbein Principle*

Prolonged high insulin levels set off a multitude of chain reactions that disrupt all other hormones and biochemical reactions at the cellular level. This chronic disruption, termed "accelerated metabolic aging," leads to body-fat gain, chronic conditions and degenerative diseases. Factors that raise insulin levels, both directly and indirectly are: eating a low-fat, high-carbohydrate diet, stress, dieting, caffeine, alcohol, aspartame (an artificial sweetener), tobacco, steroids, stimulant and other recreational drugs, lack of exercise, excessive and/or unnecessary thyroid replacement therapy and all over-the-counter and prescription drugs. These factors have become central in the eating and lifestyle habits that have prevailed over the last twenty years and that parallel the rise in the incidence of disease during this same period of time.

The Schwarzbein program, which includes balanced nutrition, stress management, exercise, the elimination of stimulants and other drugs, and hormone replacement therapy, if needed, is a complete program designed to balance insulin and all other hormone levels. Anyone can prevent accelerated aging and disease, achieve ideal body composition and extend longevity by following this program.

In addition to drastically limiting fats from our diets, since the industrial revolution most people have stopped eating foods found in nature. People now eat invented, chemically altered or created substances we call "products." We tend to think that our bodies will simply process anything we put in them. But every single thing that goes into our mouths should be used as building material or energy. If it is not, it is perceived by our bodies as a dangerous substance. Products like saccharine, margarine and other invented substances, along with refined and processed foods, are harmful to human physiology. Because chemical processes proceed on a molecular level, we must think about what we put into our bodies. In fact, since we have personally stopped eating foods found in nature, we must think about what we ingest even more.

To keep up the replenishing process within the human body, proteins and fats are the most important of the essential nutrient groups. In addition to making structures (bones, nails, hair), proteins and fats are necessary for the formation of all the chemicals needed for survival, such as hormones, enzymes and neurotransmitters. Nonstarchy vegetables are useful as a source of vitamins, minerals and fiber. Carbohydrates are used mainly to fuel the body, like gasoline for a car. Besides providing these materials and energy, *the four nutrient groups need to be eaten together to balance all the hormone systems of the body.*

Balanced Nutrition

The healing-and-maintenance eating programs (explained in detail in *The Schwarzbein Principle*) are not just one more fad diet that advocates eliminating one or two of the nutrient groups. You should not stop eating carbohydrates, or even drastically reduce carbohydrates in your diet. *This is not a high-fat, high-protein, low-carbohydrate diet.* It is a balanced nutritional program tailored to improve each individual's specific metabolism. Not eating enough carbohydrates is just as harmful as eating too many. The key to this program is determining your individual carbohydrate need. To do this *you must eat from the four basic nutrient groups* and *you must eat the quantity of real carbohydrates (not man-made) that match your activity level, current health and metabolism.*

Most people want to make healthy changes when they understand what they need to do to become healthier. However, many people either do not know how to cook, do not like to cook or do not have time to cook. With that in mind, we decided to go beyond the meal plans included in *The Schwarzbein Principle* and provide readers with easily accessible recipes to launch a new healthy lifestyle. We looked for an experienced chef who could compile our cookbooks. Evelyn Jacob Jaffe, who had culinary expertise in preparing "Schwarzbein" meals, was a natural choice. The main objective was to provide recipes that would enable readers to prepare balanced meals using real food. We all agree that Evelyn succeeded in creating and compiling healthy, delicious recipes that will motivate those who are out of the practice of preparing meals and also be easy enough for inexperienced cooks. We owe a debt of gratitude to "The Schwarzbein Principle Chef," Evelyn Jacob Jaffe, who not only has an innate sense about food and a talent for cooking but who also met the challenge of this project with a can-do attitude and a high degree of professionalism.

This cookbook is the perfect guide for all of you who want to follow The Schwarzbein Program.

Bon Appetit!

Diana Schwarzbein, M.D.
Nancy Deville

Before You Begin Cooking

Eat Enough Food

Be sure to eat as much protein, fat and nonstarchy vegetables as you want. However, everyone needs a different amount of carbohydrates depending on current health, metabolism and activity level. The recipes in this book are both for those on the Healing Program and the Maintenance Program. Carbohydrate grams vary from recipe to recipe.

It is very important to eat enough food. When you reduce your carbohydrate consumption, you *must* increase proteins, fats and non-starchy vegetables. Eating enough food is the only way to heal your metabolism and get off the accelerated metabolic aging track.[1]

Combine Recipes to Create Balanced Meals

It is important to balance your meals with proteins, fats, nonstarchy vegetables and carbohydrates. Some of the recipes in this book contain a higher amount of carbohydrates than some people should eat at one meal. To eat a balanced diet of all the essential nutrient groups, you must combine recipes. For example, if a recipe contains too

---

[1]*Accelerated metabolic aging is explained in detail in* The Schwarzbein Principle.

many carbohydrates for you, then reduce the serving size and eat it along with a main-course protein dish.

Nutritional Analysis

To help you prepare balanced meals, each recipe in this book has been analyzed and is accompanied by an approximate breakdown of protein and carbohydrate grams. These totals do not necessarily account for every carbohydrate present in each ingredient. The reason is that some recipes contain foods, such as nonstarchy vegetables, that have a low glycemic index so you can eat as much of them as you want.[2] Heavy cream, butter and other good fats also alter the glycemic index and therefore lower the number of carbohydrates in some recipes. You may notice that some recipes containing nonstarchy vegetables still show some carbohydrate. The reason is these recipes contain an ingredient, such as tomato paste, that has a higher glycemic index.

Occasionally a recipe will list a food, such as brown rice, that will not be included in the serving portion analysis. In this case, the analysis of that food will be noted separately. If not noted, then all ingredients were analyzed to come up with protein and carbohydrate grams per serving.

Fat grams are not included in the analysis, both because you should not count fat grams, and more important, you should eat as much good fat as your body needs.

Why You Do Not Need to Salt Your Foods

Our recipes do not call for salt because natural foods contain enough sodium. Eating excess salt unnecessarily strains your kidneys, contributing to the accelerated metabolic aging process. If you desire

---

[2]*The glycemic index is explained in detail in* The Schwarzbein Principle.

optimal health, you must slowly wean yourself from using salt. As you decrease your salt intake you may go through an adjustment period while you become used to the taste of food without added salt. Eventually you will be able to fully appreciate the *real* taste of food. And, more important, you will be one step closer to your goal of optimal health and an ideal body composition.

A Few Other Helpful Tips

- It is essential that you read *The Schwarzbein Principle* to fully understand the importance of a balanced diet comprised of all the essential nutrient groups: proteins, fats, nonstarchy vegetables and carbohydrates.

- Be sure to check cream containers so that you buy "all-dairy" cream. Avoid using cream or any other product containing chemical additives.

- Use real, unsalted butter. Never eat margarine or any other hydrogenated fat.

- Always buy the freshest foods possible. Use foods in their whole state—real foods that you could, in theory, pick, gather, hunt, fish or milk from an animal. Whenever possible, buy organically grown produce and grains.

- Always use whole plain yogurt and whole sour cream. Do not use low-fat or any other processed food products.

- Use only pure-pressed oils. Use mayonnaise made from pure-pressed oil.

- A few recipes call for small amounts of cornstarch and flour, which is a processed food and should not be eaten regularly.
- Occasionally you will see a recipe that calls for small amounts of orange juice. Juices are high in carbohydrates and should always be consumed as part of a balanced meal.
- Some recipes call for small amounts of alcohol. While alcohol is a stimulant and should be avoided, you can use small amounts in recipes because most of the alcohol evaporates during cooking.
- If you purchase sauces or any other products, make sure to check for sugar-free, chemical-free products.
- Buy lean meats. Lean meats contain less fat that will be damaged in the cooking process. Lean meats also contain less glycogen (sugar).
- Cook all meats over low heat to avoid damaging the fat contained in the meat.
- Before preparing recipes that contain tofu, read "All You Need to Know About Tofu" on page 291.
- Some of our recipes call for low-sodium tamari soy sauce, which does contain some salt and therefore should be used sparingly.
- Thoroughly wash all vegetables and fruits before using.
- To clean mushrooms, wipe them with a damp cloth.
- To sliver fresh basil, remove leaves from stems, rinse in cold water, roll leaves into a cigar-like tube and cut into fine slivers. (This process avoids bruising the delicate leaves.)
- To finely mince fresh ginger, peel ginger with a sharp knife or peeler, cut into thin slices and finely mince.
- If you are concerned about salmonella, do not use the recipes that call for raw eggs.

Breakfast Entrées

Assorted Entrées

Frittatas and Fabulous Variations

Omelets

Scrambled Eggs

Smoothies

Assorted Entrées

Annette Matrisciano's Cheesy Eggs

Makes 2 servings • Each serving: 25 grams protein • 2 grams carbohydrate

4 eggs

3 ounces cream cheese, cut into
½-inch cubes

¼ cup grated Parmesan cheese

freshly ground black pepper,
to taste

1½ tablespoons unsalted butter

1 minced garlic clove

In a small bowl, beat eggs with cream-cheese cubes, Parmesan cheese and black pepper. Set aside.

In a nonstick skillet, melt butter over medium-high heat. When butter is hot and bubbly, add garlic and sauté about half a minute. Pour egg mixture into skillet. Stir and fold gently until cream cheese is melted and eggs are cooked to your liking. Serve immediately.

Bacon and Eggs

Makes 2 servings • Each serving: 22 grams protein • trace carbohydrate

6 slices nitrate-free bacon	4 eggs
2 tablespoons unsalted butter	freshly ground black pepper, to taste

In a medium skillet, cook bacon over *low heat* until crisp. Remove from pan and blot dry on paper towels.

Wipe skillet clean. Melt butter over medium-high heat. When butter is hot and bubbly, crack eggs into pan. Fry 2 to 3 minutes, until whites are firm and yolks are cooked to your liking. Season to taste with black pepper.

Always cook bacon and other fatty meats over low heat to avoid damaging the fat contained in the meat. (See chapter 27 of *The Schwarzbein Principle* for a complete explanation of damaged fats.)

Breakfast Burritos

Makes 4 servings • Each serving: 17 grams protein • 17 grams carbohydrate
(Nutritional information does not include salsa)

1 tablespoon unsalted butter

2 tablespoons minced red onion

1 small minced fresh jalapeño pepper; or 1 to 2 tablespoons canned diced green chilies, to taste [wear rubber gloves to prepare fresh jalapeño pepper]

8 eggs

freshly ground black pepper, to taste

¼ teaspoon dried oregano

4 slices nitrate-free bacon, cooked and crumbled

½ cup grated Monterey Jack cheese

Topping

4 corn tortillas

¼ cup whole sour cream

½ diced ripe avocado

1 tablespoon chopped fresh cilantro

⅓ cup salsa (see Salsas, starting on page 374), or store-bought (no sugar added)

In a medium nonstick skillet, melt butter over medium-high heat. When butter is hot and bubbly, add onion and chilies and cook until softened, about 5 minutes.

In a medium bowl, using a fork, whisk eggs, black pepper and oregano until well blended. Pour eggs into skillet with onion and chilies, and cook, stirring gently, until eggs begin to set, about 2 minutes. Add crumbled bacon and grated cheese, and cook until eggs are firm. Remove from heat.

Heat tortillas by placing them one at a time over an open flame and turning with tongs until puffed up and softened; or layer tortillas between paper towels and microwave on high for 10 to 20 seconds until heated and puffed up.

Spoon ¼ of prepared mixture in center of each tortilla. Add sour cream, avocado and fresh cilantro. Fold tortillas in half and serve with salsa on the side.

Breakfast Strata

Makes 6 servings • Each serving: 25 grams protein • 30 grams carbohydrate
To reduce carbohydrate grams use a lower-carbohydrate bread.

3 tablespoons softened unsalted
butter

8 slices whole-grain bread, crusts
removed

2 cups diced nitrate-free ham

1 cup sliced brown or white
mushrooms

1 cup artichoke hearts, canned
in water, drained and
chopped

1 tablespoon chopped fresh
parsley

½ pound grated mozzarella
cheese

8 eggs

1 cup all-dairy heavy cream

¾ cup water

1 tablespoon Dijon mustard

freshly ground black pepper,
to taste

Butter both sides of bread and arrange on bottom of a greased 9 x 13-inch baking pan, cutting bread, if necessary, to fit snugly inside pan. Sprinkle diced ham over bread, followed by mushrooms, artichoke hearts and parsley. Top with grated cheese.

In a small bowl, using a fork, beat eggs with cream, water, mustard and black pepper. Pour egg mixture over bread. Cover and chill several hours or overnight. Bring to room temperature. Preheat oven to 350°. Bake strata 1 hour. Let sit 5 minutes before slicing.

Creamy Eggs Baked in Individual Ramekins, with Variations

Makes 2 servings • Each serving: 19 grams protein • trace carbohydrate

1 tablespoon unsalted butter	*freshly ground black pepper,*
4 eggs	*to taste*
2 tablespoons grated Parmesan	*¼ cup all-dairy heavy cream*
cheese	

Preheat oven to 325°. Lightly butter two 8-ounce ramekins. Crack 2 eggs into each ramekin, being careful not to break yolks. Sprinkle with Parmesan cheese. Season to taste with black pepper. Pour 2 tablespoons cream over each ramekin.

Place ramekins on a baking sheet. Bake 10 to 20 minutes, or until set to your liking.

Variations

Florentine Eggs: Into 2 buttered ramekins, divide ¾ cup cooked, drained and chopped spinach. Top with eggs, Parmesan cheese, black pepper and cream. Bake as above.

Makes 2 servings • Each serving: 20 grams protein • trace carbohydrate

Denver Eggs: Into 2 buttered ramekins, divide 1 cup cooked diced ham, or crumble 4 bacon slices. Top with eggs, Parmesan cheese, black pepper and cream. Bake as above.

Makes 2 servings • Each serving with ham: 33 grams protein • trace carbohydrate
Each serving with bacon: 23 grams protein • trace carbohydrate

Crustless Quiche, with Variations

Makes 6 servings • Each serving: 10 grams protein • trace carbohydrate

4 eggs
1 cup all-dairy heavy cream
½ cup water
freshly ground black pepper,
  to taste

dash cayenne pepper
1 cup grated Gruyère, mozzarella
  or Monterey Jack cheese

Preheat oven to 350°. In a medium bowl, using a fork, whisk eggs, cream, water, black pepper and cayenne pepper until well blended. Add grated cheese and mix well.

Butter a 9- or 10-inch pie pan. Pour in the egg and cheese mixture. Place pie pan on a baking sheet and bake 45 to 50 minutes, or until a knife inserted into center comes out clean. Let cool 5 minutes before slicing.

Variations

Bacon or Ham: Crumble 1 cup cooked nitrate-free bacon or diced nitrate-free ham into the bottom of a buttered pie pan. Cover with egg and cheese mixture and bake as above.

Makes 6 servings • Each serving with bacon: 13 grams protein • trace carbohydrate
Each serving with ham: 15 grams protein • trace carbohydrate

Spinach and Herbs: Combine 1 cup cooked, drained and chopped spinach and 2 teaspoons dried basil and spread on the bottom of a buttered pie pan. Cover with egg and cheese mixture and bake as above.

Makes 6 servings • Each serving: 11 grams protein • trace carbohydrate

Mushroom and Herbs: Combine 2 cups sautéed mixed mushrooms (shitake, oyster, brown cremini) and 1 teaspoon dried thyme and spread on the bottom of a buttered pie pan. Cover with egg and cheese mixture and bake as above. Remove from oven and sprinkle with 2 tablespoons grated Parmesan cheese.

Makes 6 servings • Each serving: 11 grams protein • trace carbohydrate

Crabmeat and Onions: Combine 6 ounces canned crabmeat (drained and picked over) and ¼ cup minced scallions and spread on the bottom of a buttered pie pan. Cover with egg and cheese mixture and bake as above. Sprinkle chopped parsley over top before serving.

Makes 6 servings • Each serving: 16 grams protein • trace carbohydrate

Eggs Benedict

Makes 4 servings • Each serving: 18 grams protein • 13 grams carbohydrate
To reduce carbohydrate grams use a lower-carbohydrate bread instead of English muffin.

4 slices nitrate-free ham or nitrate-free Canadian bacon

1 tablespoon white vinegar

8 eggs

2 whole-grain English muffins cut in halves

Classic Blender Hollandaise Sauce

In a skillet, cook ham or bacon over low heat until lightly crisped. Remove from pan and blot with paper towels.

In a deep skillet, bring 2 inches of water and vinegar to a boil over high heat. Reduce heat to simmer. Crack eggs, one at a time, into a small bowl and tip gently into boiling water. Repeat with all eggs. Cover skillet and cook 3 minutes for soft yolks, 5 minutes for firmer yolks. Using a slotted spoon, remove eggs from water and drain thoroughly.

Toast English muffins. Arrange cooked ham or bacon on top of muffins, followed by poached eggs. Top with Classic Blender Hollandaise sauce.

Classic Blender Hollandaise Sauce

3 egg yolks*

2 tablespoons fresh lemon juice

dash cayenne pepper

4 ounces (1 stick) unsalted butter, melted and bubbling hot

In a blender, combine egg yolks, lemon juice and cayenne pepper and blend on high for 3 seconds. Remove lid and, with motor running, slowly pour hot butter in a steady stream over eggs. When butter is all poured in, blend an additional 5 seconds. Taste and adjust seasonings. Serve immediately or keep sauce warm by placing blender in a bowl of warm water.

---

*If you are concerned about using raw egg, choose an alternate recipe.

Greek Eggs

Makes 2 servings • Each serving: 28 grams protein • 3 grams carbohydrate

*1 bunch spinach equal to about
1 cup cooked spinach, well
drained and chopped; or
8 ounces packaged frozen
spinach, thawed, drained
and chopped*

4 eggs

*1 tablespoon all-dairy heavy
cream*

*freshly ground black pepper,
to taste*

1½ tablespoons unsalted butter

2 tablespoons chopped red onion

1 minced garlic clove

2 teaspoons dried oregano

½ cup crumbled feta cheese

Wash spinach well, removing stems. With water still clinging to leaves, place in a medium saucepan with a tight-fitting lid. Turn heat to medium-high and steam until leaves are wilted, about 2 to 3 minutes. Drain in a colander, pressing out all liquid with the back of a wooden spoon. Chop coarsely and set aside.

In a medium bowl, using a fork, whisk eggs, cream and black pepper. In a 10-inch nonstick skillet, melt butter over medium-high heat. When butter is hot and bubbly, add onion and garlic and cook until softened, about 5 minutes. Add spinach, oregano and egg mixture. Reduce heat to medium. Cook, stirring slowly, folding eggs gently toward center of pan until cooked to your liking. Crumble in feta cheese and cook until heated through. Serve immediately.

Huevos Rancheros

Makes 4 servings • Each serving: 28 grams protein • 27 grams carbohydrate
(Nutritional information does not include salsa)

Ranchero Sauce

1 tablespoon pure-pressed
extra virgin olive oil

½ cup chopped red onion

1 minced garlic clove

½ cup canned red enchilada sauce

½ cup Basic Tomato Sauce
(recipe, page 378), or store-
bought (no sugar added); or
½ cup chopped fresh tomatoes

½ teaspoon dried oregano

1 teaspoon chili powder

¼ teaspoon ground cumin

freshly ground black pepper,
to taste

2 tablespoons chopped fresh
cilantro

8 eggs

4 corn tortillas

1 cup grated Monterey Jack
cheese

Topping

1 sliced ripe avocado

⅓ cup whole sour cream

4 sprigs fresh cilantro

½ cup salsa (see Salsas starting
on page 374), or store-bought

In a medium saucepan, heat oil over medium-high heat. When oil
is hot, add onion and garlic and cook until softened, about 5 minutes.
Add enchilada sauce, tomato sauce or tomatoes, oregano, chili powder, cumin and black pepper. Mix well. Simmer, uncovered, 10 minutes, stirring occasionally. Add chopped cilantro.

Cook eggs over-easy.

Dip tortillas into heated ranchero sauce briefly to soften and warm.
Remove from sauce and put on plates. Top with cooked eggs. Add a layer
of cheese, followed by more ranchero sauce which will melt the cheese.

Add avocado slices, sour cream and cilantro sprigs. Serve with salsa
on the side.

Oatmeal with Butter and Cream

Makes 2 servings • Each serving: 6 grams protein • 27 grams carbohydrate

Because oatmeal is high in carbohydrates, eat it as a side dish, along with a protein (eggs for example), as part of a balanced meal.

1¾ cups water

1 cup oats

2 tablespoons unsalted butter

2 tablespoons all-dairy heavy cream

In a small saucepan, bring water to a boil. Stir in oats and simmer over low heat 3 to 5 minutes, stirring occasionally. Cover pan, remove from heat and let stand until thickened, about 2 minutes. Use more water for a thinner oatmeal. Serve with butter and cream.

Poached Eggs au Gratin

Makes 2 servings • Each serving: 19 grams protein • trace carbohydrate

1 tablespoon white vinegar

4 eggs

2 tablespoons grated Parmesan cheese

2 teaspoons chopped fresh parsley

In a deep medium skillet, bring 2 inches of water and vinegar to a boil over high heat. Reduce heat to simmer. Crack an egg into a small bowl and tip gently into boiling water. Repeat with all eggs. Cover skillet and cook 3 minutes for soft yolks, 5 minutes for firmer yolks. Using a slotted spoon, remove eggs from water and drain thoroughly. Sprinkle with grated Parmesan cheese and fresh parsley. Serve immediately.

Sausage and Eggs Over-Easy

Makes 2 servings • Each serving: 34 grams protein • trace carbohydrate

6 nitrate-free turkey, beef or pork
   sausages
1½ tablespoons unsalted butter

4 eggs
freshly ground black pepper,
   to taste

In a medium nonstick skillet, cook sausages over low heat, turning occasionally, until well browned. Remove from pan and blot dry on paper towels.

In a clean nonstick skillet, melt butter over medium-high heat. When butter is hot and bubbly, crack eggs into pan. Cook 2 to 3 minutes until whites are firm and yolks are still soft. Flip eggs with a spatula and continue cooking another 30 seconds, until yolks are set to your liking. Season to taste with black pepper.

Frittatas and Fabulous Variations

Frittatas are best known in Italy. These open-faced omelets are cooked in a flameproof skillet then placed briefly under a broiler to puff up and brown.

Basic Frittata

Makes 2 servings • Each serving: 24 grams protein • trace carbohydrate

4 eggs

2 tablespoons all-dairy heavy cream

2 teaspoons minced fresh herbs (parsley, dried thyme, basil, dried oregano, dill)

freshly ground black pepper, to taste

dash cayenne pepper

2 tablespoons unsalted butter

½ cup grated mozzarella cheese

Preheat broiler. In a medium bowl, using a fork, whisk eggs, cream, fresh herbs, black pepper and cayenne pepper. Set aside.

In a 10-inch flameproof skillet, melt butter over medium-high heat. When butter is hot and bubbly, add egg mixture. As eggs cook, lift edges to allow uncooked egg to seep underneath. When bottom is set but top is still moist, spread cheese over egg and place under broiler. Broil 1 to 2 minutes, checking frequently, until top is golden and puffed up.

Avocado and Cream Cheese Frittata

Makes 2 servings • Each serving: 22 grams protein • 9 grams carbohydrate

4 eggs

2 tablespoons all-dairy heavy cream

freshly ground black pepper, to taste

dash cayenne pepper

1 tablespoon unsalted butter

Filling

1 small diced red onion

1 minced garlic clove

1½ tablespoons unsalted butter

3 tablespoons cream cheese, cut into small cubes

1 sliced ripe avocado, for topping

Preheat broiler. In a medium bowl, using a fork, whisk eggs, cream, black pepper and cayenne pepper. Set aside.

In a nonstick skillet, melt 1 tablespoon butter over medium-high heat. When butter is hot and bubbly, add onion and garlic and sauté until softened, about 5 minutes. Set aside.

In a 10-inch flameproof skillet, melt 1½ tablespoons butter over medium-high heat. When butter is hot and bubbly, add egg mixture. As eggs cook, lift edges to allow uncooked egg to seep underneath. When bottom is set but top is still moist, place cream-cheese cubes and onion mixture over eggs and place under broiler. Broil 1 to 2 minutes, checking frequently, until top is golden and puffed up. Top with sliced avocado.

Bacon, Mushroom and Artichoke Hearts Frittata

Makes 2 servings • Each serving: 26 grams protein • 8 grams carbohydrate

4 eggs

2 tablespoons all-dairy heavy cream

freshly ground black pepper, to taste

dash cayenne pepper

2 tablespoons unsalted butter

Filling

4 slices nitrate-free bacon

2 tablespoons unsalted butter

2 cups sliced brown or white mushrooms

½ cup diced artichoke hearts

1 teaspoon minced fresh rosemary, or any other fresh herb

1 tablespoon unsalted butter

2 tablespoons grated Parmesan cheese

Preheat broiler. In a medium bowl, using a fork, whisk eggs, cream, black pepper and cayenne pepper. Set aside.

In a skillet, cook bacon over low heat. Drain, blot with paper towels, crumble and set aside.

Wipe skillet clean. Melt 2 tablespoons butter over medium-high heat. When butter is hot and bubbly, add mushrooms and cook until softened and liquid is absorbed, about 5 to 7 minutes. Add artichoke hearts, rosemary or other herb and crumbled bacon. Mix well and set aside.

In a 10-inch flameproof skillet, melt remaining butter over medium-high heat. When butter is hot and bubbly, add egg mixture. As eggs cook, lift edges to allow uncooked egg to seep underneath. When bottom is set but top is still moist, spread bacon filling over egg and place under broiler. Broil 1 to 2 minutes, checking frequently, until top is golden and puffed up. Sprinkle with Parmesan cheese.

Cottage Cheesy Frittata

Makes 2 servings • Each serving: 28 grams protein • 2 grams carbohydrate

4 eggs

2 tablespoons all-dairy heavy
cream

freshly ground black pepper,
to taste

dash cayenne pepper

2 tablespoons unsalted butter

Filling

1 bunch spinach equal to about
1 cup cooked spinach, well
drained and chopped; or
8 ounces packaged frozen
spinach, thawed, drained
and chopped

½ cup whole cottage cheese

2 tablespoons grated Parmesan
cheese

2 tablespoons slivered fresh basil,
or 2 teaspoons dried basil

Preheat broiler. In a medium bowl, using a fork, whisk eggs, cream, black pepper and cayenne pepper. Set aside.

Wash spinach well, removing stems. With water still clinging to leaves, place in a medium saucepan with a tight-fitting lid. Turn heat to medium-high and cook until leaves are wilted, about two minutes. Drain in a colander, pressing out all liquid with the back of a wooden spoon. Chop and set aside.

In a small bowl combine cottage cheese, Parmesan cheese, spinach and basil. Mix well with a fork until blended. Set aside.

In a 10-inch flameproof skillet, melt butter over medium-high heat. When butter is hot and bubbly, add egg mixture. As eggs cook, lift edges to allow uncooked egg to seep underneath. When bottom is set but top is still moist, spread filling over eggs and place under broiler. Broil 1 to 2 minutes, checking frequently, until top is golden and puffed up.

Mushroom and Artichoke Hearts Frittata

Makes 2 servings • Each serving: 22 grams protein • 5 grams carbohydrate

4 eggs

2 tablespoons all-dairy heavy
cream

freshly ground black pepper,
to taste

dash cayenne pepper

Filling

2 tablespoons unsalted butter

2 cups sliced brown or white
mushrooms

½ cup artichoke hearts canned
in water, drained and chopped

1 teaspoon minced fresh rosemary,
or *any other fresh herb*

2 tablespoons unsalted butter

2 tablespoons grated Parmesan
cheese

Preheat broiler. In a medium bowl, using a fork, whisk eggs, cream, black pepper and cayenne pepper. Set aside.

In a 10-inch flameproof skillet, melt 2 tablespoons butter over medium-high heat. When butter is hot and bubbly, add mushrooms and sauté until softened, about 5 minutes. Add artichoke hearts and herbs and cook until heated through. Drain excess liquid and set aside.

In the same pan, melt 2 tablespoons butter over medium-high heat. When butter is hot and bubbly, add egg mixture. As eggs cook, lift edges to allow uncooked egg to seep underneath. When bottom is set but top is still moist, spread filling over eggs. Sprinkle with Parmesan cheese and place under broiler. Broil 1 to 2 minutes, checking frequently, until top is golden and puffed up.

Roasted Pepper and Chèvre (Goat Cheese) Frittata

Makes 2 servings • Each serving: 22 grams protein • 2 grams carbohydrate

4 eggs

2 tablespoons all-dairy heavy cream

freshly ground black pepper, to taste

dash cayenne pepper

Filling

1 red bell pepper or ¼ cup store-bought roasted red bell peppers

2 ounces fresh chèvre (goat cheese), crumbled

1 tablespoon slivered fresh basil, or 1 teaspoon dried basil

2 tablespoons chopped raw pecans

1 teaspoon grated lemon zest

2 tablespoons unsalted butter

Preheat broiler. In a medium bowl, using a fork, whisk eggs, cream, black pepper and cayenne pepper. Set aside.

If using a fresh red bell pepper, roast whole pepper directly over a gas flame or under preheated broiler on a broiler rack. Using tongs, turn pepper frequently until blistered and blackened on all sides. Place peppers in a bowl with a plate on top. Let steam for 15 minutes. Peel off all charred skin. Discard skin and seeds. Cut roasted flesh into slivers.

In a small bowl, combine slivered red bell pepper, goat cheese, basil, pecans and lemon zest. Set aside.

In a 10-inch flameproof skillet, melt butter over medium-high heat. When butter is hot and bubbly, add egg mixture. As eggs cook, lift edges to allow uncooked egg to seep underneath. When bottom is set but top is still moist, spread chèvre filling over egg mixture and place under broiler. Broil 1 to 2 minutes, checking frequently, until top is golden and puffed up.

Sausage and Onion Frittata

Makes 2 servings • Each serving: 25 grams protein • trace carbohydrate

4 eggs

2 tablespoons all-dairy heavy
cream

freshly ground black pepper,
to taste

dash cayenne pepper

1 tablespoon unsalted butter

Filling

3 nitrate-free sausage links

2 tablespoons unsalted butter

½ cup diced onion

2 teaspoons chopped fresh
rosemary, or ½ teaspoon dried
rosemary

Preheat broiler. In a medium bowl, using a fork, whisk eggs, cream, black pepper and cayenne pepper. Set aside.

Crumble sausage links into a hot skillet and cook over low heat until meat is well done. Remove from pan and set aside.

In a 10-inch flameproof skillet, melt 2 tablespoons butter over medium-high heat. When butter is hot and bubbly, sauté onion until softened, about 5 minutes. Add cooked sausage and rosemary, and mix well. Remove from pan and set aside.

In the same skillet, melt 1 tablespoon butter over medium-high heat. When butter is hot and bubbly, add egg mixture. As eggs cook, lift edges to allow uncooked egg to seep underneath. When bottom is set but top is still moist, spread sausage filling over eggs and place under broiler. Broil 1 to 2 minutes, checking frequently, until top is golden and puffed up.

Spanish-Style Tortilla Española Frittata

Makes 2 servings • Each serving: 21 grams protein • 26 grams carbohydrate

4 eggs

*2 tablespoons all-dairy heavy
  cream*

*freshly ground black pepper,
  to taste*

dash cayenne pepper

2 tablespoons unsalted butter

Filling

*2 tablespoons pure-pressed extra
  virgin olive oil*

½ cup diced onion

1 minced garlic clove

*1 large cooked and diced baking
  potato (peeled, if desired)*

*2 tablespoons grated Parmesan
  cheese*

*1 tablespoon minced fresh parsley,
  for garnish*

paprika, for garnish

Preheat broiler. In a medium bowl, using a fork, whisk eggs, cream, black pepper and cayenne pepper. Set aside.

In a 10-inch flameproof skillet, heat oil over medium-high heat. When oil is hot, add onion and garlic and sauté until softened, about 5 minutes. Add potato and stir until heated through. Remove from pan and set aside.

In the same pan, melt butter over medium-high heat. When butter is hot and bubbly, add egg mixture. As eggs cook, lift edges to allow uncooked egg to seep underneath. When bottom is set but top is still moist, spread potato filling over eggs. Sprinkle top with Parmesan cheese and place under broiler. Broil 1 to 2 minutes, checking frequently, until top is golden and puffed up. Sprinkle with parsley and paprika.

Spicy Chicken Frittata

Makes 2 servings • Each serving: 30 grams protein • trace carbohydrate

4 eggs

2 tablespoons all-dairy heavy
   cream

freshly ground black pepper,
   to taste

dash cayenne pepper

2 tablespoons unsalted butter

Filling

2 tablespoons unsalted butter

½ cup diced red bell pepper

¼ cup diced red onion

1 raw skinless, boneless chicken
   breast, diced

1 teaspoon cumin

1 teaspoon dried oregano

½ cup diced green olives

1 tablespoon grated Parmesan
   cheese

2 teaspoons finely chopped fresh
   parsley or cilantro, for garnish

Preheat broiler. In a medium bowl, using a fork, whisk eggs, cream, black pepper and cayenne pepper. Set aside.

In a 10-inch flameproof skillet, melt 2 tablespoons butter over medium-high heat. When butter is hot and bubbly, add bell peppers, onion, diced chicken, cumin, oregano and olives. Sauté about 5 minutes until chicken is tender. Remove from pan and set aside.

In the same skillet, melt remaining 2 tablespoons butter over medium-high heat. When butter is hot and bubbly, add egg mixture. As eggs cook, lift edges to allow uncooked egg to seep underneath. When bottom is set but top is still moist, spread chicken filling over egg and place under broiler. Broil 1 to 2 minutes, checking frequently, until top is golden and puffed up. Sprinkle with Parmesan cheese. Sprinkle with finely chopped parsley or cilantro.

Omelets

Chicken Liver and Onion Omelet

Makes 2 servings • Each serving: 30 grams protein • trace carbohydrate

4 eggs

2 tablespoons all-dairy heavy
cream

freshly ground black pepper,
to taste

2 tablespoons unsalted butter

Filling

2 tablespoons unsalted butter

½ cup diced onion

¼ pound rinsed and dried
chicken livers

In a medium bowl, using a fork, whisk eggs, cream and black pepper. Set aside.

In a 10-inch nonstick skillet, melt 2 tablespoons butter over medium-high heat. When butter is hot and bubbly, add onion and sauté until softened, about 5 minutes. Add chicken livers and sauté until cooked to your liking. Remove from pan, drain and set aside.

In the same skillet, melt remaining 2 tablespoons butter over medium-high heat. When butter is hot and bubbly, add egg mixture, reduce heat to medium and cook, lifting edges to allow uncooked egg to seep underneath.

When bottom layer of egg is cooked but top is still moist, spread chicken liver filling over one side of the omelet. Gently fold omelet in half. Cook half a minute longer. Slide omelet onto a plate and serve immediately.

Cream Cheese and Avocado Omelet

Makes 2 servings • Each serving: 22 grams protein • 12 grams carbohydrate

4 eggs

*2 tablespoons all-dairy heavy
cream*

*freshly ground black pepper,
to taste*

*3 ounces cream cheese, cut into
½-inch cubes*

2 tablespoons unsalted butter

Filling

1 diced ripe avocado

1 small diced tomato

*1 tablespoon minced fresh chives;
or 1 tablespoon finely chopped
scallions*

In a medium bowl, using a fork, whisk eggs, cream and black pepper. Add cream-cheese cubes and mix well. In a 10-inch nonstick skillet, melt butter over medium-high heat. When butter is hot and bubbly, add egg mixture, reduce heat to medium and cook, lifting edges to allow uncooked egg to seep underneath.

In a medium bowl, combine avocado, tomato and chives or scallions. When bottom layer of egg is cooked but top is still moist, spread avocado filling over one side of the omelet. Gently fold omelet in half. Cook half a minute longer. Slide omelet onto a plate and serve immediately.

Curried Shrimp Omelet

Makes 2 servings • Each serving: 28 grams protein • 2 grams carbohydrate

4 eggs

2 tablespoons all-dairy heavy
   cream

freshly ground black pepper,
   to taste

2 tablespoons unsalted butter

Filling

½ cup cooked small baby shrimp

¼ cup whole sour cream

1 teaspoon curry powder

2 tablespoons finely chopped
   scallions

In a medium bowl, using a fork, whisk eggs, cream and black pepper. Set aside.

In another bowl, combine shrimp, sour cream, curry powder and scallions. Set aside.

In a 10-inch nonstick skillet, melt butter over medium-high heat. When butter is hot and bubbly, add egg mixture, reduce heat to medium and cook, lifting edges to allow uncooked egg to seep underneath.

When bottom layer of egg is cooked but top is still moist, spread shrimp filling over one side of the omelet. Gently fold omelet in half. Cook half a minute longer. Slide omelet onto a plate and serve immediately.

Deli Omelet

Makes 2 servings • Each serving: 31 grams protein • 2 grams carbohydrate

4 eggs

2 tablespoons all-dairy heavy
   cream

freshly ground black pepper,
   to taste

2 tablespoons unsalted butter

Filling

½ cup diced nitrate-free ham

½ cup grated Swiss cheese, or
   provolone cheese

In a medium bowl, using a fork, whisk eggs, cream and black pepper. Set aside.

In a 10-inch nonstick skillet, melt butter over medium-high heat. When butter is hot and bubbly, add egg mixture, reduce heat to medium and cook, lifting edges to allow uncooked egg to seep underneath.

When bottom layer of egg is cooked but top is still moist, spread ham and cheese over one side of the omelet. Gently fold omelet in half. Cook half a minute longer or until cheese is melted. Slide omelet onto a plate and serve immediately.

Greek Omelet

Makes 2 servings • Each serving: 28 grams protein • 3 grams carbohydrate

4 eggs

2 tablespoons all-dairy heavy cream

freshly ground black pepper, to taste

dash cayenne pepper

2 tablespoons unsalted butter

Filling

1 bunch spinach equal to about 1 cup cooked spinach, well drained and chopped; or 8 ounces packaged frozen spinach, thawed, drained and chopped

1 tablespoon unsalted butter

2 tablespoons red onion

½ cup crumbled feta cheese

2 teaspoons dried oregano

In a medium bowl, using a fork, whisk eggs, cream and black pepper. Set aside.

Wash spinach well, removing stems. With water still clinging to leaves, place in a medium saucepan with a tight-fitting lid. Turn heat to medium-high and steam until leaves are wilted, about 2 to 3 minutes. Drain in a colander, pressing out all liquid with the back of a wooden spoon. Chop fine and set aside.

In a 10-inch nonstick skillet, melt 1 tablespoon butter over medium-high heat. When butter is hot and bubbly, add onion and sauté until softened, about 5 minutes. Remove from pan and set aside.

In a small bowl, combine sautéed onion, feta cheese, spinach and oregano.

In the same pan, melt 2 tablespoons butter over medium-high heat. When butter is hot and bubbly, add egg mixture, reduce heat to medium and cook, lifting edges to allow uncooked egg to seep underneath.

When bottom layer of egg is cooked but top is still moist, spread spinach filling over one side of the omelet. Gently fold in half. Cook half a minute longer. Slide omelet onto a plate and serve immediately.

Mushroom and Gorgonzola Omelet with Walnuts

Makes 2 servings • Each serving: 23 grams protein • 3 grams carbohydrate

4 eggs

2 tablespoons all-dairy heavy
cream

freshly ground black pepper,
to taste

Filling

2 tablespoons unsalted butter

1 cup thinly sliced brown or
white mushrooms

¼ cup finely chopped scallions

2 tablespoons crumbled
Gorgonzola, or any other blue-
veined cheese

2 tablespoons slivered fresh basil,
or 2 teaspoons dried basil

¼ cup chopped raw walnuts

In a medium bowl, using a fork, whisk eggs, cream and black pepper.
Set aside.

In a 10-inch nonstick skillet, melt butter over medium-high heat.
When butter is hot and bubbly, add sliced mushrooms and scallions
and sauté, stirring occasionally, until softened and most of liquid has
evaporated, about 5 minutes.

Add beaten egg mixture to mushrooms and scallions and cook over
medium heat until eggs begin to set. Lift edges to allow uncooked egg
to seep underneath. When bottom layer of egg is cooked but top is still
moist, spread crumbled Gorgonzola, basil and walnuts over one side
of omelet. Gently fold in half. Cook half a minute longer to melt
cheese. Slide omelet onto a plate and serve immediately.

Salmon and Caper Omelet

Makes 2 servings • Each serving: 31 grams protein • 2 grams carbohydrate

4 eggs

2 tablespoons all-dairy heavy
  cream

freshly ground black pepper,
  to taste

Filling

½ cup boned, cooked and flaked
  salmon (fresh or canned)

1 tablespoon drained and rinsed
  capers

2 teaspoons minced fresh dill, or
  1 teaspoon dried dill

¼ cup whole sour cream

2 tablespoons unsalted butter

In a medium bowl, using a fork, whisk eggs, cream and black pepper. Set aside.

In a small bowl, mix salmon, capers, dill and sour cream. Set aside.

In a 10-inch nonstick skillet, melt butter over medium-high heat. When butter is hot and bubbly, add egg mixture, reduce heat to medium and cook, lifting edges to allow uncooked egg to seep underneath.

When bottom layer of egg is cooked but top is still moist, spread salmon filling over one side of the omelet. Gently fold the omelet in half. Cook half a minute longer. Slide omelet onto a plate and serve immediately.

Spinach and Brie Omelet

Makes 2 servings • Each serving: 31 grams protein • trace carbohydrate

4 eggs

2 tablespoons all-dairy heavy
cream

freshly ground black pepper,
to taste

Filling

1 bunch spinach equal to about
1 cup cooked spinach, well
drained and chopped; or
8 ounces packaged frozen
spinach, thawed, drained
and chopped

2 tablespoons unsalted butter

2 tablespoons diced red onion

¼ pound finely sliced Brie cheese

1 tablespoon slivered fresh basil,
or 1 teaspoon dried basil

In a medium bowl, using a fork, whisk eggs, cream and black pepper.
Set aside.

Wash spinach well, removing stems. With water still clinging to
leaves, place in a medium saucepan with a tight-fitting lid. Turn heat
to medium-high and steam until leaves are wilted, about 2 to 3 minutes. Drain in a colander, pressing out all liquid with the back of a
wooden spoon. Chop and set aside.

In a 10-inch nonstick skillet, melt butter over medium-high heat.
When butter is hot and bubbly, add onion and cook until softened,
about 3 to 5 minutes. Add egg mixture, reduce heat to medium and continue cooking, lifting edges to allow uncooked egg to seep underneath.

When bottom layer of egg is cooked but top is still moist, arrange
Brie cheese slices on one side of omelet. Spread cooked spinach over
cheese and sprinkle with fresh or dried basil. Gently fold omelet in
half. Cook half a minute longer or until cheese melts. Slide omelet
onto a plate and serve immediately.

Sun-Dried Tomato and Chèvre (Goat Cheese) Omelet

Makes 2 servings • Each serving: 25 grams protein • 7 grams carbohydrate

4 eggs

2 tablespoons all-dairy heavy
cream

freshly ground black pepper,
to taste

Filling

¼ cup slivered sun-dried
tomatoes, packed in olive oil
and drained (reserve oil)

3 tablespoons crumbled chèvre
(goat cheese)

2 tablespoons finely slivered fresh
basil, or 2 teaspoons dried basil

3 tablespoons diced green olives

In a medium bowl, using a fork, whisk eggs, cream and black pepper. Set aside.

Combine sun-dried tomatoes with crumbled goat cheese, basil and green olives. Set aside.

In a 10-inch nonstick skillet, pour in 2 tablespoons of drained olive oil from sun-dried tomatoes. When oil is hot, pour in egg mixture. Cook over medium-high heat until eggs begin to set. Lift edges to allow uncooked egg to seep underneath. When bottom layer of egg is cooked but top is still moist, spread sun-dried tomato and cheese mixture over one side of omelet. Gently fold omelet in half. Cook half a minute longer until filling is hot. Slide omelet onto a plate and serve immediately.

Turkey or Pork Sausage and Cheese Omelet

Makes 2 servings • Each serving with turkey sausage: 32 grams protein • trace carbohydrate
Each serving with pork sausage: 31 grams protein • trace carbohydrate

4 eggs

2 tablespoons all-dairy heavy
cream

freshly ground black pepper,
to taste

Filling

2 tablespoons unsalted butter

½ cup diced onion

1 minced garlic clove

1 teaspoon dried oregano

¼ pound nitrate-free sausage,
removed from casings and
crumbled

¼ cup grated Monterey Jack
cheese

In a medium bowl, using a fork, whisk eggs, cream and black pepper.
Set aside.

In a 10-inch nonstick skillet, melt butter over medium-high heat.
When butter is hot and bubbly, add onion and garlic and sauté until
softened, about 5 minutes. Add oregano and sausage and sauté until
sausage is browned. Drain fat from pan.

Reduce heat to medium, add egg mixture and continue cooking,
lifting edges to allow uncooked egg to seep underneath. Cook until
eggs are set and bottom is lightly browned. Add grated cheese. Gently
fold omelet in half and cook half a minute longer or until cheese
melts. Slide omelet onto a plate and serve immediately.

Western Omelet

Makes 2 servings • Each serving: 23 grams protein • trace carbohydrate

4 eggs

*2 tablespoons all-dairy heavy
cream*

*freshly ground black pepper,
to taste*

Filling

2 tablespoons unsalted butter

3 tablespoons diced onion

½ diced green bell pepper

½ cup diced nitrate-free ham

*2 tablespoons chopped fresh
parsley, for garnish*

In a medium bowl, using a fork, whisk eggs, cream and black pepper. Set aside.

In a 10-inch nonstick skillet, melt butter over medium-high heat. When butter is hot and bubbly, add onion and bell pepper. Cook until softened, about 5 minutes. Add ham and cook another 2 minutes.

Reduce heat to medium, add egg mixture and cook, lifting edges to allow uncooked egg to seep underneath. Continue cooking until eggs are set and bottom is lightly browned. Gently fold omelet in half. Top with parsley and slide onto a plate. Serve immediately.

Scrambled Eggs

Basic Scrambled Eggs

Makes 2 servings • Each serving: 16 grams protein • trace carbohydrate

4 eggs
2 tablespoons all-dairy heavy
cream

freshly ground black pepper,
to taste
2 tablespoons unsalted butter

In a medium bowl, using a fork, whisk eggs, cream and black pepper. Set aside.

In a 10-inch nonstick skillet, melt butter over medium-high heat. When butter is hot and bubbly, add eggs to pan. Reduce heat to medium. Gently stir egg mixture around with a wooden spoon, stirring until eggs are soft, creamy and cooked to your liking. Serve immediately.

Asian Scramble

Makes 2 servings • Each serving: 40 grams protein • trace carbohydrate

4 eggs

2 tablespoons all-dairy heavy
cream

freshly ground black pepper,
to taste

2 tablespoons pure-pressed
peanut oil

2 tablespoons minced scallions

2 tablespoons minced fresh
cilantro

1 teaspoon peeled and finely
minced fresh ginger

¼ cup thinly sliced celery stalks

1 cup sliced brown or white
mushrooms

1 cup medium raw shrimp,
shelled and deveined

2 teaspoons low-sodium tamari
soy sauce

In a small bowl, using a fork, whisk eggs, cream and black pepper.
Set aside.

In a 10-inch nonstick skillet, heat oil over medium-high heat. When
oil is hot, add scallions, cilantro, ginger, celery, mushrooms and
shrimp, and sauté until shrimp turns pink, about 5 minutes. Drain
excess liquid from pan. Add soy sauce and mix well. Add egg mixture
and gently stir with a wooden spoon until cooked to your liking. Serve
immediately.

Bacon Scramble

Makes 2 servings • Each serving: 28 grams protein • trace carbohydrate

4 eggs

2 tablespoons all-dairy heavy
cream

freshly ground black pepper,
to taste

4 slices nitrate-free bacon

2 tablespoons unsalted butter

1 diced tomato

½ cup grated mozzarella cheese

In a small bowl, using a fork, whisk eggs, cream and black pepper.
Set aside.

In a 10-inch nonstick skillet, cook bacon over low heat until crisp.
Drain on paper towels. Crumble and set aside.

In a 10-inch nonstick skillet, melt butter over medium-high heat.
When butter is hot and bubbly, add egg mixture. Gently stir egg mixture with a wooden spoon. Add crumbled bacon, tomato and cheese
and continue stirring until cheese melts and eggs are cooked to your
liking. Serve immediately.

Deli Scramble

Makes 2 servings • Each serving: 23 grams protein • trace carbohydrate

4 eggs

2 tablespoons all-dairy heavy
cream

freshly ground black pepper,
to taste

2 tablespoons unsalted butter

½ cup diced onion

½ cup diced nitrate-free ham

In a small bowl, using a fork, whisk eggs, cream and black pepper. Set aside.

In a 10-inch nonstick skillet, melt butter over medium-high heat. When butter is hot and bubbly, add onion and sauté until softened, about 5 minutes. Add egg mixture and ham. Gently stir egg mixture with a wooden spoon until cooked to your liking. Serve immediately.

San Francisco Joe's Special
(scrambled eggs, hamburger meat and spinach)

Makes 2 servings • Each serving: 49 grams protein • trace carbohydrate

*1 bunch spinach equal to about
1 cup cooked spinach, well
drained and chopped; or
8-ounce package frozen
spinach, thawed, drained
and chopped*

½ pound lean hamburger meat

2 tablespoons unsalted butter

½ cup chopped onion

1 minced garlic clove

¼ teaspoon dried oregano

*freshly ground black pepper,
to taste*

4 eggs

*2 tablespoons grated Parmesan
cheese*

Wash spinach well, removing stems. With water still clinging to leaves, place in a medium saucepan with a tight-fitting lid. Turn heat to medium-high and steam until leaves are wilted, about 2 to 3 minutes. Drain in a colander, pressing out all liquid with the back of a wooden spoon. Chop coarsely and set aside.

In a medium skillet, cook hamburger over medium heat until browned, breaking apart lumps with a wooden spoon. Remove meat from pan, drain fat and set aside.

In a large nonstick skillet, melt butter over medium-high heat. When butter is hot and bubbly, add onion, garlic, oregano and black pepper and sauté until softened, about 5 minutes. Add spinach and hamburger meat and stir until spinach is heated through.

In a small bowl, using a fork, beat eggs and pour over meat mixture. Gently move egg/meat mixture around with a wooden spoon until cooked to your liking. Sprinkle with Parmesan cheese. Taste, and adjust seasonings. Serve immediately.

Santa Barbara Scrambled Eggs

Makes 2 servings • Each serving: 23 grams protein • 3 grams carbohydrate

4 eggs

2 tablespoons all-dairy heavy cream

freshly ground black pepper, to taste

2 tablespoons unsalted butter

1 cup sliced brown or white mushrooms

3 ounces cream cheese, cut into ½-inch cubes

2 tablespoons grated Parmesan cheese

2 tablespoons slivered fresh basil, or 1 teaspoon dried basil

1 tablespoon minced fresh parsley

In a medium bowl, using a fork, whisk eggs, cream and black pepper. Set aside.

In a 10-inch nonstick skillet, melt butter over medium-high heat. When butter is hot and bubbly, add sliced mushrooms. Cook until mushrooms are softened, about 5 minutes. Drain excess liquid.

Pour beaten egg mixture over mushrooms. Reduce heat to medium. Gently stir egg mixture with a wooden spoon, about 1 minute. Sprinkle cream cheese, Parmesan cheese, basil and parsley evenly over eggs. Continue folding until cheese is melted and eggs are set. Serve immediately.

South of the Border Scramble

Makes 2 servings • Each serving: 21 grams protein • 19 grams carbohydrate

4 eggs

2 tablespoons all-dairy heavy
cream

freshly ground black pepper,
to taste

2 tablespoons unsalted butter

½ diced red onion

½ diced bell pepper

1 small diced fresh jalapeño
pepper; or 1 tablespoon
canned diced green chilies
[wear rubber gloves to
prepare fresh jalapeño pepper]

½ cup corn

1 diced medium tomato

2 tablespoons chopped fresh
cilantro

Topping

1 sliced ripe avocado

2 tablespoons whole sour cream

2 sprigs fresh cilantro

In a small bowl, using a fork, whisk, eggs, cream and black pepper.
Set aside.

In a 10-inch nonstick skillet, melt butter over medium-high heat.
When butter is hot and bubbly, add onion, bell pepper and jalapeño
pepper and sauté until softened, about 5 minutes. Add corn, tomato,
cilantro and egg mixture. Gently stir egg mixture with a wooden
spoon until cooked to your liking. Arrange eggs on a plate and top
with avocado, sour cream and cilantro sprigs. Serve immediately.

Smoothies

If a recipe is high in carbohydrates, it should not be eaten alone as a meal. Instead combine it with a higher-protein recipe to create a balanced meal.

Peanut Butter Smoothie with Yogurt and Banana

Makes 1 smoothie • 13 grams protein • 28 grams carbohydrate

½ cup whole plain yogurt

2 tablespoons organic peanut butter, chunky or smooth (no honey or sugar added)

½ banana

2 crushed ice cubes

Combine all ingredients in a blender. Blend on high until smooth and creamy.

Peanut Butter Smoothie
with Yogurt and Dates

Makes 1 smoothie • 13 grams protein • 29 grams carbohydrate

½ cup whole plain yogurt

2 tablespoons organic peanut
butter, chunky or smooth
(no honey or sugar added)

2 pitted dates

2 crushed ice cubes

Combine all ingredients in a blender. Blend on high until smooth and creamy.

Yogurt Smoothie
with Cottage Cheese and Strawberries

Makes 1 smoothie • 12 grams protein • 13 grams carbohydrate

½ cup whole plain yogurt

¼ cup whole cottage cheese

4 strawberries, sliced

2 crushed ice cubes

Combine all ingredients in a blender. Blend on high until smooth and creamy.

Appetizers, Snacks, Dips and Spreads

Appetizers and Snacks with Chicken

Appetizers and Snacks with Meat

Appetizers and Snacks Without Meat

Appetizers and Snacks with Seafood

Dips

Spreads

Appetizers and Snacks with Chicken

Chicken Saté with Peanut Sauce

Makes 4 servings • Each serving: 30 grams protein • 2 grams carbohydrate

1 pound skinless, boneless
chicken breasts

2 tablespoons smooth organic
peanut butter (no honey or
sugar added)

1 tablespoon low-sodium tamari
soy sauce

1 tablespoon fresh lime juice

1 teaspoon peeled and finely
minced fresh ginger

1 minced garlic clove

2 teaspoons chopped fresh cilantro

dash cayenne pepper

eight 8-inch bamboo skewers
soaked in water 15 minutes to
prevent burning

Preheat oven to 450°. Rinse chicken under cold water and pat dry with paper towels. Cut chicken into 1½-inch pieces.

In a blender or food processor, blend peanut butter, soy sauce, lime juice, ginger, garlic, cilantro and cayenne pepper until smooth. Taste, and adjust seasonings. Coat chicken with peanut sauce marinade and marinate, refrigerated, 30 minutes or longer.

Thread about 6 pieces of chicken on each skewer. Arrange skewers on a greased rack with a tinfoil-lined baking sheet underneath. Bake until fully cooked, turning occasionally, about 7 to 10 minutes. Place under broiler for the last 2 minutes to brown, turning once. Transfer to a serving plate and serve hot.

(To serve with dipping sauce, double peanut sauce marinade and reserve half. Heat the dipping sauce before serving.)

Mint Pesto Chicken Kabobs

Makes 6 servings • Each serving: 30 grams protein • trace carbohydrate

*1½ pounds skinless, boneless
chicken breasts*

Mint Pesto

2 cups loosely packed mint leaves

½ cup loosely packed fresh basil

*½ cup loosely packed fresh
cilantro*

¼ cup grated Parmesan cheese

2 minced garlic cloves

2 tablespoons fresh lime juice

*½ cup pure-pressed extra virgin
olive oil*

*freshly ground black pepper,
to taste*

dash cayenne pepper

*twelve 8-inch wooden skewers
soaked in water 15 minutes
to prevent burning*

Preheat oven to 400°. Rinse chicken under cold water and pat dry
with paper towels. Cut chicken into 1½-inch pieces. In a blender or
food processor, blend pesto ingredients until mixed well. Taste, and
adjust seasonings.

Coat chicken pieces with pesto paste and marinate, refrigerated, 15
minutes or longer. Thread 3 to 5 chunks of chicken onto each skewer.
Arrange skewers on a greased rack with a tinfoil-lined baking sheet
underneath. Bake until chicken is fully cooked, turning occasionally,
about 7 to 10 minutes. Place under broiler for last 2 minutes to brown,
turning once. Transfer to a serving plate and serve hot.

Pecan Chicken Salad

Makes about 1 ½ cups • Each ¼ cup serving: 10 grams protein • 2 grams carbohydrate

¼ cup coarsely chopped raw
  pecans

2 boneless, skinless chicken
  breasts

2 bay leaves

1 tablespoon minced scallions

2 teaspoons minced fresh parsley

¼ cup finely chopped celery
  stalks

⅓ cup mayonnaise (made from
  pure-pressed oil)

1 teaspoon Dijon mustard

freshly ground black pepper,
  to taste

paprika, for garnish

Put pecans in an ungreased skillet over medium-high heat. Stir nuts or shake pan almost constantly, until pecans are evenly browned and toasted. Remove from pan immediately and set aside.

Bring 1 inch of water and bay leaves to a boil in a skillet. Reduce heat to medium. Add chicken, cover and poach until cooked through, about 20 minutes, turning once. *Do not overcook.* Let cool and shred with fingers.

In a medium bowl, using a fork, combine all ingredients except paprika. Taste, and adjust seasonings. To serve, spread on celery sticks, cucumber rounds or bell pepper squares. Sprinkle with paprika.

Sesame Chicken

Makes 4 servings • Each serving: 29 grams protein • trace carbohydrate

1 pound skinless, boneless
  chicken breasts

Marinade

1 to 2 tablespoons low-sodium
  tamari soy sauce, to taste

1 teaspoon peeled and finely
  minced fresh ginger

1 teaspoon minced garlic cloves

1 tablespoon dry sherry

2 tablespoons pure-pressed
  sesame oil

1 tablespoon minced fresh cilantro

dash cayenne pepper

2 tablespoons raw sesame seeds

Rinse chicken under cold water and pat dry with paper towels. Cut chicken into 1½-inch pieces.

In a small bowl, using a fork, combine soy sauce, ginger, garlic, sherry, sesame oil, cilantro and cayenne pepper. Mix well. Add chicken pieces and coat thoroughly. Marinate, refrigerated, at least 2 hours, turning occasionally.

Preheat oven to 450°. Remove chicken from marinade and arrange on a greased baking sheet. Sprinkle with sesame seeds and bake, uncovered, until cooked through, about 7 to 10 minutes, turning once. Broil for the last minute to brown, if desired. Serve warm, with toothpicks.

Appetizers and Snacks with Meat

Ham and Green Chile Crustless Quiche

Makes 8 servings • Each serving: 11 grams protein • trace carbohydrate

2 tablespoons unsalted butter

½ cup chopped red onion

3 tablespoons canned diced green chilies

1 cup finely diced nitrate-free ham

1 teaspoon dried oregano

freshly ground black pepper, to taste

4 eggs

1 cup all-dairy heavy cream

1 cup Swiss, Monterey Jack or mozzarella cheese

dash cayenne pepper

Preheat oven to 350°. In a large skillet, melt butter over medium-high heat. When butter is hot and bubbly, add onion and sauté until softened, about 5 minutes. Add green chilies, diced ham, oregano and black pepper. Mix well. Remove from heat and set aside.

In a medium bowl, using a fork, whisk eggs, cream, cheese and cayenne pepper. Combine with ham mixture and gently mix.

Butter an 8-inch-square pan or a 9-inch pie pan. Pour mixture into buttered pan. Bake until golden brown and puffed up, about 25 minutes. Let stand 10 minutes before slicing.

Sausage-Filled Mushrooms

Makes 6 servings • Each serving: 9 grams protein • 1 gram carbohydrate

*1 bunch spinach equal to about
1 cup cooked spinach, well
drained and chopped; or
8-ounce package frozen
spinach, thawed, drained
and chopped*

12 large stuffing mushrooms

*2 tablespoons pure-pressed extra
virgin olive oil*

*½ pound spicy or mild nitrate-
free Italian sausage*

2 tablespoons unsalted butter

½ cup chopped red onion

2 minced garlic cloves

¼ cup minced celery stalks

¼ cup chopped raw pecans

¼ teaspoon dried thyme

½ teaspoon dried dill

¼ teaspoon dried oregano

*freshly ground black pepper,
to taste*

dash cayenne pepper

*2 tablespoons grated Parmesan
cheese*

Preheat oven to 375°. Wash spinach well, removing stems. With water still clinging to leaves, place in a heavy saucepan with a tight-fitting lid. Turn heat to medium-high and steam until leaves are wilted, about 2 to 3 minutes. Drain in a colander, pressing out all liquid with the back of a wooden spoon. Chop fine and set aside.

Wipe mushrooms clean with a damp cloth. Remove stems from mushrooms and chop fine. Set aside. Using your fingers, rub tops of mushrooms with olive oil.

Crumble sausage into a hot frying pan and brown over low heat. Using a slotted spoon, transfer drained meat to a medium bowl.

In a clean skillet, melt butter over medium-high heat. When butter is hot and bubbly, add onion, garlic and celery. Sauté until softened and lightly browned, about 5 minutes. Add pecans, thyme, dill, oregano, black pepper, cayenne pepper, chopped spinach and mushroom stems. Mix well and sauté 3 minutes. Remove from heat and let mixture cool slightly. Combine with sausage in medium bowl. Taste, and adjust seasonings.

Mound a rounded tablespoon of sausage mixture into each mushroom cavity. Arrange filled mushrooms on a lightly greased baking sheet, sprinkle with Parmesan cheese and bake 15 minutes, or until heated through. Serve hot.

Savory Meatballs

Makes about 2 dozen meatballs.
Each 3-meatball serving: 16 grams protein • 5 grams carbohydrate
(Nutritional information does not include pesto mayonnaise)

1 pound lean ground beef, or
   turkey

1 beaten egg

½ cup fresh or dried whole-grain
   bread crumbs

1 minced garlic clove

¼ cup minced scallions

1 tablespoon low-sodium tamari
   soy sauce

1 tablespoon Dijon mustard

freshly ground black pepper,
   to taste

Pesto Mayonnaise

Preheat oven to 450°. In a large bowl, using a fork or wooden spoon, combine all ingredients, except Pesto Mayonnaise, blending well. Using your hands, form the meat mixture into 1-inch balls. Arrange meatballs on a lightly greased baking sheet so that they do not touch. Bake until browned and fully cooked, turning occasionally to brown evenly, about 10 to 12 minutes. (Prepared meatballs can be frozen uncooked; *or* covered and refrigerated 1 day before cooking.) Transfer to a serving dish and serve with Pesto Mayonnaise.

Pesto Mayonnaise

Makes about 1½ cups. Each 2 tablespoon serving: 6 grams protein • 2 grams carbohydrate

1 cup mayonnaise (made from
   pure-pressed oil)

½ cup Pesto (see Pestos, starting
   on page 371), or store-bought
   (no sugar added)

In a small bowl, using a whisk or fork, blend mayonnaise and pesto. Transfer to a dipping bowl and serve with meatballs.

Appetizers and Snacks Without Meat

Artichokes with Hollandaise Sauce

Makes 4 servings • Each serving: 6 grams protein • 13 grams carbohydrate

4 artichokes

1 quartered lemon

Classic Blender Hollandaise Sauce

With a sharp knife, slice off top of each artichoke and trim stems so that they sit upright. Use kitchen shears to trim points off ends of leaves. Place artichokes in 4 inches of boiling water along with a quartered lemon. Boil uncovered, about 35 to 45 minutes, or until leaves pull away easily and are tender.

Serve with Classic Blender Hollandaise Sauce on the side, in dipping bowls.

Classic Blender Hollandaise Sauce

3 egg yolks*

2 tablespoons fresh lemon juice

dash cayenne pepper

4 ounces (1 stick) unsalted butter melted and bubbling hot

In a blender, combine egg yolks with lemon juice and cayenne pepper, on high for 3 seconds. Remove lid and, with motor running, slowly pour hot butter in a steady stream over eggs. When butter is all poured in, blend an additional 5 seconds. Taste, and adjust seasonings. Serve immediately or keep sauce warm by placing blender in a bowl of warm water.

Makes about 1 cup.

---

*If you are concerned about using raw egg, choose an alternate recipe.

Asparagus Spears in Garlic Vinaigrette

Makes 4 servings • Each serving: trace protein • trace carbohydrate

1 pound asparagus, tough ends
   trimmed

Garlic Vinaigrette

2 tablespoons balsamic vinegar

2 minced garlic cloves

1 teaspoon Dijon mustard

freshly ground black pepper,
   to taste

⅓ cup pure-pressed extra virgin
   olive oil

1 tablespoon grated Parmesan
   cheese

In a large skillet, bring 1 inch of water to a boil over medium-high heat. Add asparagus and cook until tender, about 3 to 6 minutes. Remove from pan, drain and arrange on a serving platter.

In a blender or food processor, blend all vinaigrette ingredients until smooth; or place ingredients in a jar with a tight-fitting lid and shake vigorously until well blended. Pour over asparagus and serve at room temperature.

Cheesy Quesadillas

Makes 8 servings • Each serving: 9 grams protein • 20 grams carbohydrate
(Nutritional information does not include salsa)

Filling

2 tablespoons canned diced green
   chilies

¼ cup minced scallions

1 tablespoon pure-pressed
   monounsaturated vegetable oil
   or *unsalted butter*

2 tablespoons minced fresh
   cilantro

1½ cups grated Monterey Jack
   cheese

8 corn tortillas

Toppings

2 thinly sliced ripe avocados

1 cup whole sour cream

½ cup *Papaya* or *Mango Salsa*
(*see recipe, page 375*)

In a medium bowl, combine filling ingredients.

In a medium nonstick skillet, heat oil or butter over medium-high heat. When hot, add a corn tortilla and heat on one side before flipping over. Spoon ¼ cup of filling on half of tortilla. Do not overfill. Fold plain half of tortilla over.

Cook each side about 2 to 3 minutes, until cheese is melted and filling is hot. Add more oil or butter to pan as needed and cook remaining tortillas the same way. Add sliced avocado and sour cream before serving. Serve salsa on the side.

Curried Deviled Eggs

Makes 12 halves • Each half: 4 grams protein • trace carbohydrate

6 hard-boiled eggs

4 tablespoons mayonnaise
(made from pure-pressed oil)

2 teaspoons Dijon mustard

1 teaspoon curry powder

cayenne pepper, to taste

2 tablespoons chopped fresh
cilantro, or parsley, for garnish

paprika, for garnish

To hard boil eggs, place eggs in a medium saucepan and cover with cold water. Bring to a boil uncovered. Allow to boil for 1 minute, then cover, remove from heat and let sit undisturbed 10 minutes. Rinse eggs under cold water. Crack shells, peel and rinse eggs.

Cut peeled eggs in half lengthwise. Carefully remove yokes and put into a medium bowl. Add remaining ingredients, except cilantro/parsley and paprika. Mash with a fork until smooth. Taste, and adjust seasonings.

Using a small teaspoon, fill egg-white cavities with about 1 tablespoon of curry mixture per egg. Sprinkle tops with cilantro or parsley and paprika. Arrange on a serving platter.

Marinated Mushrooms

Makes 4 servings • Each serving: 2 grams protein • trace carbohydrate

½ pound small brown or white
   mushrooms

3 tablespoons pure-pressed extra
   virgin olive oil

1 tablespoon water

juice of 1 lemon

½ teaspoon dried thyme

1 minced garlic clove

4 tablespoons finely chopped
   fresh parsley

freshly ground black pepper,
   to taste

Wipe mushrooms clean with a damp cloth. Trim stems and set mushrooms aside.

In a medium saucepan, bring oil, water, lemon juice, thyme, garlic and parsley to a boil. Add mushrooms and simmer 10 minutes, stirring occasionally. Season to taste with black pepper. Put mushrooms into a serving bowl and let cool. Taste, and adjust seasonings. Serve, with toothpicks on the side.

Pecan Cheese Ball

Makes 6 servings • Each serving: 9 grams protein • 3 grams carbohydrate

½ cup chopped raw pecans

8 ounces cream cheese, softened
at room temperature

4 ounces crumbled Gorgonzola
cheese, or *any other blue-
veined cheese*

2 tablespoons minced fresh
parsley

2 tablespoons slivered fresh basil,
or *1 teaspoon dried basil*

freshly ground black pepper,
to taste

Put pecans in an ungreased skillet over medium-high heat. Stir nuts or shake pan almost constantly, until pecans are evenly browned and toasted. Remove from pan immediately and set aside to cool.

In a food processor, blend softened cream cheese, Gorgonzola cheese, parsley, basil, black pepper and ¼ cup chopped, toasted pecans until smooth, breaking up any lumps with a spatula.

Form cheese mixture into a ball and place in a small bowl lined with plastic wrap. Seal and refrigerate several hours or overnight. A half hour before serving, remove from refrigerator. Unwrap and sprinkle with ¼ cup reserved pecans. Serve with assorted raw vegetables.

Salad Stix

Makes 8 servings • Each serving: 5 grams protein • 4 grams carbohydrate

16 small fresh mozzarella balls

¼ cup pure-pressed extra virgin olive oil

3 minced garlic cloves

freshly ground black pepper, to taste

2 red bell peppers, roasted and cut into large chunks, or ½ cup store-bought roasted red peppers

16 fresh basil leaves

16 marinated mushrooms, prepared (see recipe, page 71) or store-bought

8 large green olives

2 cups marinated artichoke hearts, drained and cut into chunks

eight 8-inch bamboo skewers

Drain fresh mozzarella balls and rinse with water. In a small bowl mix together oil, garlic and black pepper. Add mozzarella balls and marinate 15 minutes or overnight, if possible.

If using fresh red bell peppers, roast peppers directly over a gas flame, or under preheated broiler on a broiler rack. Using tongs, turn peppers frequently until blistered and blackened on all sides. Place peppers in a bowl with a plate on top. Let steam for 15 minutes to loosen skins. Peel off all charred skin. Discard skin along with seeds. Cut roasted flesh into 1-inch pieces.

Take a bamboo skewer and put on a mozzarella ball moving it down to the base of the stick. Next put on a whole basil leaf followed by a red bell pepper chunk, mushroom, green olive, artichoke heart, basil leaf, red bell pepper chunk, mushroom and mozzarella ball. Repeat with other sticks until all ingredients have been used up.

Arrange on a platter and serve immediately.

Sesame Baked Mushrooms

Makes about 20 mushrooms • Each mushroom: 1 gram protein • 2 grams carbohydrate

¼ cup raw sesame seeds

1 pound medium brown or white
mushrooms

1 beaten egg

1 teaspoon Dijon mustard

freshly ground black pepper,
to taste

¼ cup fresh or dried whole-grain
bread crumbs

Put sesame seeds in an ungreased skillet over medium-high heat. Stir seeds or shake pan almost constantly until seeds are lightly browned and begin to pop. Remove from pan immediately and set aside.

Preheat oven to 350°. Wipe mushrooms clean with a damp cloth. Trim stems and set mushrooms aside. In a small bowl, using a fork, mix beaten egg with mustard and black pepper. In a separate bowl, mix sesame seeds and bread crumbs.

Spear stem end of mushrooms with a fork. Dip cap into egg mixture, then into bread-crumb mixture. Place on a greased rack with a tinfoil-lined baking sheet underneath. Bake 15 to 20 minutes, until golden brown. Serve hot.

Spicy Mixed Nuts

Makes about 4 cups • Each ¼ cup serving: 6 grams protein • 7 grams carbohydrate

3 tablespoons pure-pressed extra
   virgin olive oil

2 minced garlic cloves

1 teaspoon low-sodium tamari
   soy sauce

½ teaspoon ground cumin

1 teaspoon curry powder

dash red-pepper flakes

½ teaspoon chili powder

1 cup whole raw almonds

1 cup whole raw cashews

1 cup raw pecan halves

1 cup whole raw peanuts

Preheat oven to 350°. In a large skillet, heat oil over medium heat. When oil is hot, add garlic and sauté until softened, about 10 seconds. Add soy sauce, cumin, curry powder, red-pepper flakes and chili powder. Stir well. Add mixed nuts and stir until thoroughly coated with spices.

Transfer nut mix to a baking sheet. Bake 15 to 20 minutes, stirring frequently to bake evenly. Remove from oven and cool. Store in an airtight container.

Spinach-and-Cheese-Stuffed Mushrooms

Makes 6 servings • Each serving: 10 grams protein • 3 grams carbohydrate

1 bunch spinach equal to about 1 cup cooked spinach, well drained and chopped; or 8 ounces packaged frozen spinach, thawed, drained and chopped

12 large stuffing mushrooms

2 tablespoons unsalted butter

2 tablespoons minced scallions

1 minced garlic clove

1 cup whole ricotta or whole cottage cheese

¼ cup grated Parmesan cheese

2 tablespoons slivered fresh basil, or 1 teaspoon dried basil

freshly ground black pepper, to taste

2 tablespoons pure-pressed extra virgin olive oil

2 tablespoons grated Parmesan cheese

paprika, for garnish

Preheat oven to 375°. Wash spinach well, removing stems. With water still clinging to leaves, place in a medium saucepan with a tight-fitting lid. Turn heat to medium-high and steam until leaves are wilted, about 2 to 3 minutes. Drain in a colander, pressing out all liquid with the back of a wooden spoon. Chop fine and set aside.

Wipe mushrooms clean with a damp cloth. Remove stems and chop fine. Set caps aside. In a skillet, melt butter over medium-high heat. When butter is hot and bubbly, add scallions, garlic and chopped mushroom stems and sauté until softened, about 5 minutes. Remove from heat and put into a large bowl along with drained spinach, ricotta or cottage cheese, Parmesan cheese, basil and black pepper. Mix well with a wooden spoon. Taste, and adjust seasonings.

Using your fingers, lightly oil tops of mushroom caps. Mound each mushroom cavity with about 1 tablespoon of filling. Arrange mushrooms, cavity-side up, on a greased rack with a tinfoil-lined baking sheet underneath. Sprinkle with Parmesan cheese and paprika. Bake until thoroughly heated, about 15 to 20 minutes. Serve hot.

Appetizers and Snacks with Seafood

Caviar Pie

Makes 8 servings • Each serving: 11 grams protein • 2 grams carbohydrate

8 hard-boiled eggs

¼ cup mayonnaise (made from pure-pressed oil)

2 teaspoons Dijon mustard

freshly ground black pepper, to taste

1 cup whole sour cream

2 ounces black caviar

½ cup finely chopped fresh parsley

⅓ cup finely chopped red onion

½ cup finely chopped scallions

½ cup finely chopped red bell pepper, or 4 ounces red pimentos, drained well and chopped

To hard boil eggs, place eggs in a saucepan and cover with cold water. Bring to a boil uncovered. Allow to boil for 1 minute then cover, remove from heat and let sit undisturbed for 10 minutes. Rinse eggs under cold water. Crack shells, peel and rinse eggs.

Chop eggs and combine with mayonnaise, mustard and black pepper, mixing well. Spread egg mixture evenly across bottom of a lightly greased 9-inch glass pie pan or comparable glass dish. Stir sour cream with a fork until creamy. Spread sour cream smoothly over egg mixture, completely covering top.

Mound caviar into the center of pie. Surround caviar with a ring of parsley followed by a ring of chopped red onion and another ring of chopped scallions. Form a final ring of chopped bell pepper or pimentos. Serve with assorted cut-up raw vegetables.

Ceviche

Makes 6 servings • Each serving: 37 grams protein • trace carbohydrate

2 pounds very fresh raw fish
(any combination of halibut,
red snapper, scallops, flounder,
sea bass)

2 cups fresh lime juice

⅓ cup pure-pressed extra virgin
olive oil

½ cup finely chopped red onion

2 small, diced fresh red or green
hot chili peppers [wear rubber
gloves to prepare fresh chili
peppers]

2 minced garlic cloves

3 tablespoons chopped fresh
cilantro

freshly ground black pepper,
to taste

dash cayenne pepper

Remove skin and bones from fish and cut into small ½-inch pieces. In a medium bowl, combine lime juice, olive oil, red onion, chilies, garlic, cilantro, black pepper and cayenne pepper. Pour over fish and mix well. Be sure that fish is completely immersed in marinade—the lime juice "cooks" the fish. Cover and refrigerate 3 to 4 hours.

Drain almost all marinade from ceviche. Taste, and adjust seasonings. Pour into a medium serving bowl.

Crab and Artichoke Crustless Quiche

Makes 6 servings • Each serving: 17 grams protein • 6 grams carbohydrate

2 tablespoons unsalted butter

½ cup chopped shallots

1 diced red bell pepper

15 ounces artichoke hearts,
canned in water, drained and
chopped

6 ounces canned crabmeat,
drained, picked over and
chopped

2 teaspoons grated lemon zest

2 tablespoons minced fresh parsley

3 eggs

1¼ cups all-dairy heavy cream

¾ cup grated Monterey Jack
cheese, or crumbled feta cheese,
or crumbled Gorgonzola cheese

1 tablespoon grated Parmesan
cheese

freshly ground black pepper,
to taste

dash cayenne pepper

1 tablespoon grated Parmesan
cheese, for topping

1 tablespoon minced fresh parsley

Preheat oven to 350°.

In a large nonstick skillet, melt butter over medium-high heat. When butter is hot and bubbly, add shallots and bell pepper and sauté, stirring frequently until softened, about 5 minutes. Mix in chopped artichokes, crabmeat, lemon zest and 2 tablespoons parsley. Continue cooking and stirring 5 minutes. Remove from heat and set aside.

In a large bowl, using a fork, whisk eggs, cream, grated or crumbled cheese, Parmesan cheese, black pepper and cayenne pepper. Gently stir in artichoke and crab mixture. Pour filling into a buttered 8-inch square baking pan or 9-inch pie pan. Sprinkle with additional Parmesan cheese and bake until golden and puffed up, about 25 to 30 minutes. Broil top until browned and bubbly, about 30 seconds. Sprinkle with 1 tablespoon minced parsley. Let stand 10 minutes before serving.

Crabmeat Salad on Cucumber Rounds

Makes 8 servings • Each serving: 13 grams protein • 1 gram carbohydrate

8 ounces cream cheese, softened
  at room temperature

¼ cup whole sour cream

12 ounces canned crabmeat,
  drained, picked over and
  chopped

2 tablespoons fresh lemon juice

1 minced garlic clove

1 tablespoon all-dairy heavy
  cream

1 tablespoon minced red onion

1 hothouse English cucumber

1 tablespoon minced celery

1 tablespoon minced scallions

2 tablespoons finely chopped
  fresh parsley

2 teaspoons Dijon mustard

1 tablespoon drained and rinsed
  capers

freshly ground black pepper,
  to taste

dash cayenne pepper

paprika, for garnish

In a medium bowl, using a fork, mix cream cheese and sour cream until smooth. Stir in remaining ingredients, except cucumber and paprika, and mix well. Taste, and adjust seasonings. Cover and refrigerate 30 minutes.

Cut an unpeeled hothouse English cucumber into 1½-inch rounds. Using a melon-baller or small spoon, scoop out center flesh and seeds from one end of the round, leaving the other end intact. The rounds will now sit on a plate with scooped-out cavity ready for filling. Spoon a tablespoon of crabmeat salad into each cavity and dust top lightly with paprika.

Curried Tuna on Endive

Makes 12 servings • Each serving: 8 grams protein • trace carbohydrate

⅓ cup chopped raw pecans

1 to 2 teaspoons curry powder, to taste

13 ounces tuna, packed in oil or water and drained

2 tablespoons drained and rinsed capers

3 tablespoons chopped celery

3 tablespoons fresh lemon juice

2 heads endive lettuce

2 tablespoons chopped fresh parsley

2 teaspoons Dijon mustard

2 tablespoons minced scallions

⅓ cup mayonnaise (made from pure-pressed oil)

freshly ground black pepper, to taste

dash cayenne pepper

paprika, for garnish

Put pecans and curry powder in an ungreased skillet over medium-high heat. Stir nuts and curry powder or shake pan almost constantly, until pecans are evenly browned and toasted. Remove from pan immediately and set aside.

Drain tuna well. In a medium bowl, using a fork, flake tuna and add capers, celery, lemon juice, parsley, mustard, scallions, mayonnaise, curry powder, pecans, black pepper and cayenne pepper. Mix well. Taste, and adjust seasonings.

Cut root end from endive and separate leaves. Wash and dry well. Mound 1 to 2 tablespoons of tuna mixture onto each endive leaf. Sprinkle with paprika and serve.

Grandma Anne's Famous Salmon Balls

Makes 8 servings • Each serving: 16 grams protein • 2 grams carbohydrate

½ cup finely chopped raw pecans

15 ounces canned red or pink salmon, drained, picked over and flaked

8 ounces cream cheese, softened at room temperature

1 tablespoon diced red onion

1 tablespoon finely chopped fresh parsley

1 tablespoon finely chopped scallions

2 teaspoons fresh lemon juice

1 teaspoon Dijon mustard

freshly ground black pepper, to taste

dash cayenne pepper

2 tablespoons chopped fresh parsley

Put pecans in an ungreased skillet over medium-high heat. Stir nuts or shake pan almost constantly, until pecans are evenly browned and toasted. Remove from pan immediately and set aside.

In a medium bowl, using a fork, combine salmon and softened cream cheese. Add red onion, parsley, scallions, lemon juice, mustard, black pepper and cayenne pepper and mix well. Refrigerate several hours or overnight.

Using your hands, roll salmon mixture into 1½-inch-diameter balls. Roll the balls in chopped pecans and then in parsley. Refrigerate until ready to eat.

Red Potatoes with Sour Cream and Caviar

Makes 12 caviar-filled potatoes • Each potato: 1 gram protein • 5 grams carbohydrate

6 small red potatoes

¼ cup whole sour cream

½ ounce caviar

whole sprigs fresh parsley,
   for garnish

In a medium saucepan, cover potatoes with cold water. Bring to a boil and cook until just tender, about 15 minutes. Drain and let cool. Cut potatoes in half. Cut a small slice from bottom of each half so potatoes sit flat on serving plate.

Using a small spoon or melon-baller, scoop out a ball of potato, leaving a shell of about ¼ inch. Stir sour cream and gently spoon a dollop into the cavity of each potato half. Top with caviar. Transfer to a serving plate and garnish with whole sprigs of parsley.

Seafood Paté

Makes 8 servings • Each serving: 25 grams protein • 1 gram carbohydrate

3 hard-boiled eggs, chopped

3 tablespoons unsalted butter

1 minced garlic clove

6 finely chopped scallions

½ pound scallops

½ pound raw shrimp, peeled and deveined

6 ounces canned crabmeat, drained, picked over and chopped

8 ounces cream cheese, softened at room temperature

2 tablespoons Dijon mustard

2 tablespoons horseradish

3 tablespoons fresh lime juice

2 tablespoons drained and rinsed capers

1 teaspoon paprika

dash cayenne pepper

lime slices, for garnish

To hard boil eggs, place eggs in a saucepan and cover with cold water. Bring to a boil uncovered. Allow to boil for one minute, then cover, remove from heat, and let sit undisturbed 10 minutes. Rinse eggs under cold water. Crack shells, peel and rinse eggs.

In a large nonstick skillet, melt butter over medium-high heat. When butter is hot and bubbly, add garlic, scallions and scallops. Sauté until scallops are almost tender, about 3 to 5 minutes. Add shrimp and crabmeat and sauté, stirring well, another 2 minutes, or until shrimp turn pink.

In a food processor, purée sautéed seafood with remaining ingredients until smooth. Taste and adjust seasonings. Transfer to a serving dish and garnish with lime slices. Serve with cut-up raw vegetables.

Shrimp with Spicy Cocktail Sauce

Makes 4 servings • Each serving: 29 grams protein • 1 gram carbohydrate

1 pound raw jumbo shrimp

Spicy Cocktail Sauce

⅔ cup mayonnaise (made from pure-pressed oil)

⅓ cup whole sour cream

1 teaspoon grated lime zest

1 tablespoon fresh lime juice

1 tablespoon chopped fresh cilantro or parsley

2 to 3 tablespoons chili sauce, to taste

freshly ground black pepper, to taste

In a large pot, bring 1 quart of water to a boil. Add shrimp. Reduce heat to low and simmer 2 to 3 minutes, until shrimp turn pink. Using a slotted spoon, remove from boiling water. Rinse immediately under cold water for 2 minutes. Peel shrimp and devein by slicing along back ridge with a small sharp knife and carefully lifting out the black vein. Cool to room temperature before refrigerating.

In a medium bowl, using a fork, combine all cocktail sauce ingredients. Mix well. Taste, and adjust seasonings. Cover and refrigerate. To serve, arrange shrimp in a circular pattern around a small bowl filled with cocktail sauce.

Stuffed Celery with Crab

Makes 4 servings • Each serving: 9 grams protein • 8 grams carbohydrate

½ cup sliced raw almonds,
  for garnish

1 tablespoon unsalted butter

1 teaspoon dried mustard

1 teaspoon curry powder

8 ounces cream cheese, softened
  at room temperature

2 tablespoons Apricot and Raisin
  Chutney (see recipe, page 365)
  or store-bought, (no sugar
  added)

½ cup fresh or canned crabmeat,
  drained, picked over and
  chopped

1 tablespoon fresh lime juice

cayenne pepper, to taste

4 stalks celery

paprika, for garnish

Put almonds in an ungreased skillet over medium-high heat. Stir or shake pan almost constantly, until almonds are evenly browned and toasted. Remove from pan immediately and set aside.

In a small nonstick skillet, melt butter over medium-high heat. When butter is hot and bubbly, reduce heat to medium and add dried mustard and curry powder and sauté until lightly browned, about 1 minute.

In a medium bowl, using a fork, blend cream cheese, sautéed spices, chutney, crab, lime juice and cayenne pepper. Taste, and adjust seasonings. Wash and trim celery. Cut into 2-inch lengths. Trim bottom edge of each length of celery so it will sit flat on serving plate. Spoon filling into celery cavities and sprinkle with toasted almonds.

Stuffed Roasted Bell Peppers with Shrimp, Feta Cheese and Olives

Makes 6 servings • Each serving: 18 grams protein • 3 grams carbohydrate

½ pound crumbled feta cheese

2 tablespoons lemon juice

2 tablespoons pure-pressed extra virgin olive oil

2 tablespoons finely chopped red onion

¼ cup seeded and diced cucumber

1 minced garlic clove

1 teaspoon dried oregano

¼ cup finely chopped Kalamata olives

1 cup cooked baby shrimp, diced

dash cayenne pepper

1 each red, gold and green bell peppers or ¾ cup store-bought roasted bell peppers

In a medium bowl, using a fork, combine all ingredients except bell peppers. Mix well. Taste, and adjust seasonings.

If using fresh bell peppers, roast peppers directly over a gas flame or under preheated broiler on a broiler rack. Using tongs, turn peppers frequently, until blistered and blackened on all sides. Place peppers in a bowl with a plate on top. Let steam for 15 minutes to loosen skins. Peel off all charred skin.

Slice roasted flesh into 2-inch wide strips. Spoon 1 to 2 tablespoons filling at end of each strip and roll up, jelly-roll fashion. Repeat with remaining strips and filling.

Dips

Chutney Dip

Makes about 2 cups • 2 tablespoons: 5 grams protein • 9 grams carbohydrate

¾ cup sliced raw almonds

1 pound cream cheese, softened
at room temperature

1 cup Apricot and Raisin
Chutney (see recipe, page 365)
or store-bought (no sugar
added)

2 teaspoons curry powder

½ teaspoon dried mustard

Put almonds in an ungreased skillet, over medium-high heat. Stir nuts or shake pan almost constantly, until almonds are evenly browned and toasted. Remove from pan immediately and set aside.

In a food processor, blend cream cheese with ½ cup chutney, curry powder and mustard until smooth. Spoon into a bowl lined with plastic wrap. Fold plastic wrap over dip and seal. Refrigerate at least 2 hours.

Invert bowl onto serving platter and remove plastic wrap. Pour remaining chutney over top and sides of cheese spread. Sprinkle with toasted almonds and serve with cut-up raw vegetables.

Cream Cheese Pesto Dip

Makes about 1½ cups • 2 tablespoons: 5 grams protein • 2 grams carbohydrate

½ cup Basil Pesto (see recipe, page 372) or store-bought

8 ounces cream cheese, softened at room temperature

3 whole basil leaves, for garnish

In a small bowl, using a fork, combine pesto and cream cheese, blending until smooth; or blend in a food processor until smooth. Taste, and adjust seasonings.

To serve, mound dip in a small bowl and garnish with whole basil leaves. Serve with cut-up raw vegetables.

Curried Shrimp Dip

Makes 6 servings • Each serving: 10 grams protein • 2 grams carbohydrate

8 ounces cream cheese, softened at room temperature

¼ cup whole sour cream

2 tablespoons fresh lime juice

1 cup cooked baby shrimp

1 teaspoon curry powder

3 tablespoons thinly sliced scallions

1 teaspoon peeled and finely minced fresh ginger

1 tablespoon all-dairy heavy cream

freshly ground black pepper, to taste

dash cayenne pepper

2 teaspoons minced fresh cilantro, for garnish

In a medium bowl, using a fork, combine cream cheese and sour cream, blending well. Stir in remaining ingredients, except cilantro, and mix well. Taste, and adjust seasonings. Cover and refrigerate 2 to 4 hours.

To serve, mound in a small bowl. Sprinkle with minced cilantro and surround with assorted raw vegetables.

Famous Hot Artichoke Cheese Dip

Makes 8 servings • Each serving: 7 grams protein • 5 grams carbohydrate

13 ¾ ounces canned artichoke
hearts canned in water,
drained and rinsed

8 ounces cream cheese, diced into
small cubes

⅓ cup mayonnaise (made from
pure-pressed oil)

⅔ cup grated Parmesan cheese

2 tablespoons slivered fresh basil,
or 1 teaspoon dried basil

1 teaspoon grated lemon zest

freshly ground black pepper,
to taste

dash cayenne pepper

Preheat oven to 425°. Coarsely chop drained artichoke hearts. Mix with cream cheese, mayonnaise, Parmesan cheese, basil, lemon zest, black pepper and cayenne pepper. Transfer to a lightly oiled oven-proof casserole or 9-inch pie pan and bake about 20 minutes, until hot and bubbly. Serve with cut-up raw vegetables.

Garlic Herb Dip with Toasted Walnuts

Makes about 1¼ cups • Each ¼ cup serving: 5 grams protein • 3 grams carbohydrate

½ cup chopped raw walnuts

8 ounces cream cheese, softened at room temperature

3 tablespoons fresh lemon juice

1 minced garlic clove

1 tablespoon finely chopped fresh parsley

1 teaspoon mixed dried Italian herbs (basil, oregano, thyme)

freshly ground black pepper, to taste

2 tablespoons all-dairy heavy cream

Put walnuts in an ungreased medium skillet over medium-high heat. Stir nuts or shake pan almost constantly, until walnuts are evenly browned and toasted. Remove from pan immediately and set aside.

In a food processor, purée cream cheese with lemon juice, garlic, parsley, herbs, black pepper and cream until smooth. Put into a bowl, cover and refrigerate 2 hours.

To serve, sprinkle toasted walnuts on top. Surround dip with cut-up raw vegetables.

Gorgonzola Dip

Makes about 1³/₄ cups • Each ¼ cup serving: 6 grams protein • 1 gram carbohydrate
1 small apple: 15 grams carbohydrate • 1 small pear: 17 grams carbohydrate

4 ounces Gorgonzola or *any*
other blue-veined cheese

3 ounces cream cheese, softened
at room temperature

½ cup whole sour cream

¼ cup all-dairy heavy cream

1 tablespoon fresh lime juice

2 tablespoons slivered fresh basil,
or 1 teaspoon dried basil

freshly ground black pepper,
to taste

In a food processor, purée all ingredients until smooth, or in a medium bowl, using a fork, mash Gorgonzola cheese with cream cheese. Add sour cream and heavy cream and blend until smooth. Gently mix in lime juice, basil and black pepper. Taste, and adjust seasonings. Transfer to a serving bowl, and surround with apple and pear slices and cut-up raw vegetables.

Guacamole

Makes about 2 cups • Each ¼ cup serving: 2 grams protein • 6 grams carbohydrate

3 ripe avocados

3 tablespoons minced red onion

1 minced garlic clove

2 tablespoons fresh lemon or lime juice

1 tablespoon chopped fresh cilantro

1 to 2 tablespoons salsa (see Salsas, starting on page 374), or store-bought, (no sugar added) or a few drops hot-pepper sauce

freshly ground black pepper, to taste

Cut avocados in half. Remove pits and scoop flesh into a medium bowl. Mash with a fork. Add remaining ingredients and mix well. Taste, and adjust seasonings.

Insert 1 avocado pit into mixture to prevent pulp from turning brown. Store covered in refrigerator. To serve, remove pit, mound in a small serving bowl and surround with cut-up raw vegetables.

Hummus

Makes about 2½ cups • Each ¼ cup serving: 7 grams protein • 16 grams carbohydrate

2 cans (30 ounces) garbanzo
 beans, drained and rinsed

2 minced garlic cloves

4 to 6 tablespoons fresh lemon
 juice, to taste

½ cup sesame tahini

¼ cup pure-pressed extra virgin
 olive oil

¼ to ½ cup water, as needed
 to thin

½ teaspoon ground cumin

cayenne pepper, to taste

paprika

In a food processor, combine drained beans with garlic, lemon juice, sesame tahini, olive oil, water, cumin and cayenne pepper until well blended. Taste, and adjust seasonings, adding more lemon juice if desired.

To serve, mound dip in a medium serving bowl. Sprinkle with paprika and surround with cut-up raw vegetables.

Spreads

Chèvre (Goat Cheese) Spread

Makes about 2 cups • Each ¼ cup serving: 4 grams protein • 7 grams carbohydrate

1 cup sun-dried tomatoes in
olive oil

½ cup chèvre (goat cheese)

1 cup coarsely chopped green
olives

3 minced garlic cloves

2 tablespoons chopped fresh
parsley

1 teaspoon grated lemon zest

freshly ground black pepper,
to taste

In a blender or food processor, combine all ingredients, including oil from tomatoes, until smooth. Taste, and adjust seasonings. Mound dip in a small bowl and surround with cut-up raw vegetables.

Chèvre (Goat Cheese) with Pistachio Nuts

Makes about 1 cup • Each ¼ cup serving: 10 grams protein • 5 grams carbohydrate
1 small apple: 15 grams carbohydrate • 1 small pear: 17 grams carbohydrate

3 ounces chèvre (goat cheese)

3 ounces cream cheese, softened
at room temperature

1 tablespoon all-dairy heavy
cream

⅓ cup finely chopped dry-roasted
pistachio nuts

dash cayenne pepper

¼ cup chopped dry-roasted
pistachio nuts, for garnish

In a medium bowl, using a fork, blend chèvre (goat cheese), cream cheese, cream, ⅓ cup chopped pistachio nuts and cayenne pepper. Transfer to a serving bowl and top with reserved pistachio nuts.

Spread on apple and pear slices or celery sticks.

Feta Cheese Spread with Cucumber Rounds

Makes 6 servings • Each serving: 7 grams protein • 2 grams carbohydrate

½ pound crumbled feta cheese

1 tablespoon fresh lemon juice

1½ tablespoons pure-pressed extra virgin olive oil

6 finely chopped Kalamata olives

1 tablespoon finely chopped fresh parsley

1 tablespoon finely chopped red onion

2 tablespoons chopped dry-roasted pistachio nuts

freshly ground black pepper, to taste

1 hothouse English cucumber

extra whole dry-roasted pistachio nuts, for garnish

In a medium bowl, using a fork or your fingers, crumble feta cheese. Add lemon juice and olive oil and mix well. Add olives, parsley, red onion, chopped pistachio nuts and black pepper. Mix until well blended. Taste, and adjust seasonings.

Cut an unpeeled hothouse English cucumber into 1½-inch rounds. Using a melon-baller or small spoon, scoop out center flesh and seeds from one end of the round, leaving the other end intact. The rounds will now sit on a plate with a scooped-out cavity ready for filling. Spoon a tablespoon of feta filling into cavity. Garnish with a whole pistachio nut.

Pecan Baked Brie

Makes 8 servings • Each serving: 3 grams protein • trace carbohydrate
1 small apple: 15 grams carbohydrate • 1 small pear: 17 grams carbohydrate

8-ounce wheel of Brie cheese
1 tablespoon softened unsalted
  butter

¼ cup whole raw pecans

Preheat oven to 350°. Place Brie wheel in a lightly greased 8-inch glass pie pan or similar ovenproof dish. Spread butter over cheese, thoroughly covering white rind. Arrange whole pecans on top. Bake 10 to 12 minutes or until cheese begins to melt. Serve with apple and pear slices.

Quick Mushroom Paté Spread

Makes about 2 cups • Each ¼ cup serving: 2 grams protein • 3 grams carbohydrate

1 cup chopped raw walnuts

3 tablespoons unsalted butter

1 small finely chopped onion

1 minced garlic clove

½ pound chopped brown or
white mushrooms

1 tablespoon low-sodium tamari
soy sauce

freshly ground black pepper,
to taste

1 tablespoon minced fresh parsley

Put walnuts in an ungreased medium skillet over medium-high heat. Stir nuts or shake pan almost constantly until walnuts are evenly browned and toasted. Remove from pan immediately and set aside to cool.

In a large nonstick saucepan, melt butter over medium-high heat. When butter is hot and bubbly, add onion and sauté until softened, about 5 minutes. Add mushrooms and sauté until softened and tender, about 5 minutes. Drain excess liquid from pan.

Transfer to a food processor. Add walnuts, soy sauce and black pepper. Purée until smooth. Taste, and adjust seasonings. Transfer to a serving bowl, sprinkle with parsley and surround with cut-up raw vegetables.

Sun-Dried Tomato Pesto

Makes about 1 cup • Each ¼ cup serving: 9 grams protein • 14 grams carbohydrate

1 cup sun-dried tomatoes in
   olive oil

2 tablespoons slivered fresh basil,
   or 1 teaspoon dried basil

¼ cup grated Parmesan cheese

1 minced garlic clove

⅛ teaspoon red-pepper flakes

In a blender or food processor, blend tomatoes with oil from jar, basil, Parmesan cheese, garlic and red-pepper flakes until smooth. Taste, and adjust seasonings.

Transfer to a serving bowl and serve at room temperature with cut-up raw vegetables.

Virginia Farber's Famous Liver Paté

Makes 8 servings • Each serving: 14 grams protein • trace carbohydrate

¼ teaspoon unflavored gelatin

¼ cup water

¼ cup condensed beef consommé, low-sodium canned

1 pound chicken livers

1 cup softened unsalted butter

⅓ cup finely chopped onion

1 teaspoon dry mustard

¼ teaspoon ground nutmeg

1 tablespoon anchovy paste

dash cayenne pepper

dash ground cloves

fresh parsley sprigs, for garnish

Soften gelatin in water. In a small saucepan, heat consommé and softened gelatin, stirring occasionally until gelatin is completely dissolved. Pour into a 2½- to 3-cup mold. Chill until firm.

In a small saucepan, cover livers with water, bring to a boil and simmer over low heat until tender, about 8 to 10 minutes. Drain and cool slightly before transferring to a food processor along with the softened butter. Purée livers until smooth. Add onion, mustard, nutmeg, anchovy paste, cayenne pepper and cloves and process until well blended.

Spread liver mixture over consommé in the mold, gently pressing the liver mixture down evenly. Cover and chill until firm. Unmold and garnish with fresh parsley sprigs.

Whole Roasted Garlic

Makes 6 servings • Each serving: trace protein • trace carbohydrate
Check packaging for nutritional analysis of crackers or bread.

3 whole garlic bulbs

2 tablespoons pure-pressed extra
  virgin olive oil

freshly ground black pepper,
  to taste

Preheat oven to 425°. Peel off any loose outer layers of skin from whole garlic bulbs, leaving cloves intact and unpeeled. Slice off the top ½ inch of the bulbs and discard.

Drizzle bulbs with olive oil and sprinkle with black pepper. Arrange on a lightly greased baking sheet and bake until cloves are browned and bursting out of their skins, about 20 minutes. Cool slightly. Squeeze pulp out of skins and spread on low-carbohydrate whole-grain crackers or bread.

Soups

Bean and Grain Soups

Chicken Soups

Homemade Stocks

Meat Soups

Seafood Soups

Vegetable Soups

Bean and Grain Soups

To eat a balanced diet of all the essential nutrient groups, you must combine recipes. For example, if you prepare a soup that does not contain adequate protein, or contains too many carbohydrates, eat the soup as a side dish and prepare another protein dish to eat as a main course.

African Quinoa Soup with Vegetables

Makes 6 servings • Each serving: 13 grams protein • 20 grams carbohydrate

2 tablespoons unsalted butter

1 medium chopped onion

2 minced garlic cloves

1 small minced fresh jalapeño
pepper; or 1 to 2 tablespoons
canned diced green chilies,
to taste [wear rubber gloves to
prepare fresh jalapeño pepper]

1 diced red bell pepper

2 diced celery stalks with leaves

2 medium diced zucchini

1 medium diced sweet potato

1 teaspoon ground cumin

1 teaspoon dried oregano

6 cups chicken or vegetable stock
(see recipes, pages 113 and
115), or low-sodium canned

½ cup quinoa, rinsed and
drained

freshly ground black pepper,
to taste

dash cayenne pepper

½ cup chunky organic peanut
butter (no honey or sugar added)

In a large heavy-bottomed soup pot, melt butter over medium-high heat. When butter is hot and bubbly, add onion, garlic, jalapeño pepper, bell pepper, celery, zucchini, sweet potato, cumin and oregano. Sauté 10 to 15 minutes, or until vegetables are softened.

Add stock, quinoa, black pepper and cayenne pepper. Bring to a boil, reduce heat and cover. Simmer until quinoa is cooked and vegetables are tender, about 10 to 15 minutes. Add peanut butter, using a wooden spoon to blend in completely, and simmer another 10 minutes. Taste, and adjust seasonings.

Black Bean Soup

Makes 6 servings • Each serving: 7 grams protein • 20 grams carbohydrate

2 cups dried black beans, picked over, rinsed and soaked overnight

2 tablespoons pure-pressed extra virgin olive oil

1 medium chopped red onion

3 minced garlic cloves

1 diced green or red bell pepper

½ cup chopped celery

½ cup diced carrots

1 teaspoon ground cumin

1 teaspoon chili powder

1 teaspoon dried oregano

2 bay leaves

14½ ounces canned tomatoes, chopped and peeled, with juice

freshly ground black pepper, to taste

3 tablespoons finely chopped fresh cilantro

dash hot-pepper sauce (optional)

1 to 2 tablespoons fresh lime juice, to taste

½ cup whole sour cream

Soak beans overnight by covering tops of beans with at least 4 inches of water. Drain and rinse well. Place beans in a large heavy-bottomed soup pot and cover with about 10 cups of fresh water. Bring to a boil. Reduce heat to medium and cook, uncovered, until tender, about 45 minutes to 1 hour, skimming off any foam that may collect on the surface.

In a large nonstick skillet, heat oil over medium-high heat. When oil is hot, add red onion, garlic, bell pepper, celery, carrots, cumin and chili powder, and sauté until softened, about 8 minutes. Add oregano, bay leaves, tomatoes and their juice. Stir well.

Add sautéed vegetable mixture to cooked beans and mix well. Cook over low heat 30 minutes, stirring occasionally, until beans are soft. Add more water if necessary. Remove bay leaves. Season to taste with black pepper. Stir in chopped cilantro, hot-pepper sauce and lime juice. Taste, and adjust seasonings. Blend until smooth in a blender or food processor, if desired. Serve with a spoonful of sour cream.

Moroccan Curried Lentil Soup

Makes 8 servings • Each serving: 12 grams protein • 12 grams carbohydrate

3 tablespoons unsalted butter

1 large diced onion

2 minced garlic cloves

1 diced green or red bell pepper

2 diced celery stalks with leaves

2 diced carrots

2 zucchini, quartered lengthwise, then diced

1 teaspoon ground cumin

1 teaspoon ground curry powder

2 cups lentils, picked over and rinsed

8 cups chicken stock (see recipe, page 113), or low-sodium canned

1 bay leaf

1 tablespoon peeled and finely minced fresh ginger

1 cup diced tomatoes

3 tablespoons finely chopped fresh cilantro

freshly ground black pepper, to taste

1 tablespoon fresh lemon juice

In a large heavy-bottomed soup pot, melt butter over medium-high heat. When butter is hot and bubbly, add onion, garlic and bell pepper and cook until softened, about 5 minutes. Add celery, carrots, zucchini, cumin and curry powder and sauté 5 minutes. Add lentils, stock and bay leaf. Bring to a boil, reduce heat, and simmer over low heat, covered, 30 to 45 minutes, or until lentils are tender. Add ginger, tomatoes, cilantro and black pepper. Simmer another 15 minutes to blend flavors. Add lemon juice. Taste, and adjust seasonings.

Mushroom Barley Soup

Makes 6 servings • Each serving: 10 grams protein • 13 grams carbohydrate

3 tablespoons unsalted butter

1 medium chopped onion

2 minced garlic cloves

2 diced celery stalks with leaves

2 diced carrots

2 teaspoons dried oregano

1 teaspoon dried thyme

2 bay leaves

½ cup pearl barley, rinsed and drained

6 cups chicken stock (see recipe, page 113), or low-sodium canned

2 tablespoons unsalted butter

¾ pound thinly sliced brown or white mushrooms

1 cup fresh green peas or frozen and thawed

freshly ground black pepper, to taste

2 tablespoons finely chopped fresh parsley, for garnish

In a large heavy-bottomed soup pot, melt butter over medium-high heat. When butter is hot and bubbly, add onion and garlic and cook until softened, about 5 minutes. Add celery, carrots, oregano, thyme, bay leaves and barley, and stir until well blended.

Add stock and bring to a boil. Reduce heat to low. Cover and simmer until barley is tender, about 45 minutes.

In a large saucepan, melt butter over medium-high heat. When butter is hot and bubbly, add sliced mushrooms and sauté until softened and their liquid has been released, about 5 minutes. Add mushrooms to soup pot along with peas and black pepper. Simmer over low heat 5 minutes or until peas are tender. Taste, and adjust seasonings. Serve garnished with finely chopped parsley.

Chicken Soups

Anytime Soup is a "prescription" soup to eat during the initial phase of the Healing Program as described in *The Schwarzbein Principle*. If you are hungry *between meals*, eat Anytime Soup as a snack.

Anytime Soup

Makes 8 servings • Each serving: 5 grams protein • 10 grams carbohydrate

1 pound chicken parts or soup bones

½ head shredded green cabbage

1 minced garlic clove

2 chopped celery stalks

2 pounds diced fresh tomatoes

3 chopped carrots

2 tablespoons chopped fresh parsley

½ teaspoon dried thyme (optional)

½ teaspoon dried basil (optional)

freshly ground black pepper, to taste

4 cups chicken stock (see recipe, page 113), or vegetable stock (see recipe, page 115), or low-sodium canned, or 4 cups water

2 tablespoons fresh lemon juice, or 2 tablespoons cider vinegar

In a large heavy-bottomed soup pot, bring all ingredients, except lemon juice or vinegar to a boil. Lower heat and simmer 1 hour. Remove chicken parts or soup bones. Shred chicken and return to pot. Add lemon juice or vinegar. Taste, and adjust seasonings.

Chicken Corn Chowder

Makes 4 servings • Each serving: 36 grams protein • 15 grams carbohydrate

2 tablespoons unsalted butter

1 cup finely chopped shallots

2 minced garlic cloves

1 red bell pepper, diced into ¼-inch cubes

1 small finely diced fresh jalapeño pepper; or 1 to 2 tablespoons canned diced green chilies, to taste [wear rubber gloves to prepare fresh jalapeño pepper]

2 red potatoes, diced into ½-inch cubes (peeled, if desired)

1 bay leaf

4 cups chicken stock (see recipe, page 113), or vegetable stock (see recipe, page 115), or low-sodium canned

2 cups raw, diced chicken

1 cup fresh corn kernels or frozen and thawed

1 cup all-dairy heavy cream

1 tablespoon finely chopped fresh cilantro

freshly ground black pepper, to taste

dash cayenne pepper

In a large heavy-bottomed soup pot, melt butter over medium-high heat. When butter is hot and bubbly, add shallots, garlic, bell pepper and jalapeño pepper, and sauté until softened, about 5 to 8 minutes. Add potatoes, bay leaf, stock and chicken. Bring to a boil, reduce heat to low and simmer, uncovered, until potatoes and chicken are tender, about 10 minutes. Add corn, cream, cilantro, black pepper and cayenne pepper. Cook over low heat until well blended and heated through, about 5 minutes. *Do not boil.* Taste, and adjust seasonings.

Mama's "You'll Feel Better" Chicken Soup

Makes 6 servings • Each serving: 45 grams protein • 6 grams carbohydrate

2 pounds cut-up chicken parts, breasts and thighs

2 quarts chicken stock (see recipe, page 113), or low-sodium canned

1 bay leaf

1 medium chopped onion

1 well-washed, small finely chopped leek

1 minced garlic clove

3 carrots, cut diagonally into ¼-inch pieces

1 parsnip, peeled and cut diagonally into ¼-inch pieces

2 celery stalks with leaves, cut diagonally into ¼-inch pieces

¼ cup finely chopped fresh parsley

freshly ground black pepper, to taste

Rinse chicken under cold water and pat dry with paper towels. In a heavy-bottomed soup pot, bring chicken stock to a boil over medium-high heat. Add chicken and bay leaf and reduce heat to low. Cover and poach until cooked through, about 10 minutes. Remove chicken from stock, drain, and shred meat, discarding skin and bones. Set meat aside.

Add onion, leeks, garlic, carrots, parsnip and celery to soup pot. Simmer over low heat, covered, about 20 minutes until vegetables are tender. Add shredded chicken, parsley and black pepper. Taste, and adjust seasonings.

Homemade Stocks

Beef Stock

After straining, makes about 3 quarts.
Each 1 cup serving: 5 grams protein • 2 grams carbohydrate

4 pounds meaty beef or veal bones

½ to 1 bulb garlic, unpeeled and halved crosswise

2 well-washed, coarsely chopped leeks

2 large onions, peeled, quartered and studded with 8 whole cloves

4 celery stalks with leaves, cut into 2-inch pieces

2 carrots, peeled and cut into 2-inch chunks

½ pound brown or white mushrooms, quartered

3 bay leaves

12 whole black peppercorns

1 bunch coarsely chopped fresh parsley

4 to 5 sprigs fresh thyme, or 2 teaspoons dried thyme

4 quarts water

In a large heavy-bottomed soup pot, bring all ingredients to a boil. Reduce heat to low, stir well and cover. Simmer 3 to 4 hours, skimming off any foam that collects on surface.

Remove pot from heat. Allow stock to cool slightly. Using a spoon, skim excess fat from top and strain stock through a fine-meshed sieve.

Thoroughly cool before refrigerating or freezing for future use.

Chicken Stock

After straining, makes about 3 quarts.
Each 1 cup serving: 3 grams protein • 1 gram carbohydrate

1 whole stewing chicken (about 5 to 6 pounds)

4 quarts water

2 large onions, quartered and studded with 3 to 4 whole cloves

4 peeled garlic cloves

2 well-washed, coarsely chopped leeks

3 carrots, cut into 2-inch chunks

4 celery stalks with leaves, cut into 2-inch pieces

3 parsnips, cut into 2-inch chunks

1 bunch coarsely chopped fresh parsley

3 bay leaves

4 to 5 fresh sprigs thyme, or 2 teaspoons dried thyme

10 whole black peppercorns

Rinse chicken under cold water and pat dry with paper towels. Cut chicken into quarters. In a large soup pot, bring chicken and water to a boil. Skim off foam as it collects on the surface. When no more foam appears, add remaining ingredients. Bring back to a boil, reduce heat and simmer, partially covered, 2 to 4 hours. The longer the stock cooks, the richer it will taste.

Remove stock from heat, and cool. Strain stock through a fine-meshed sieve. Reserve chicken for another use. Thoroughly cool before refrigerating or freezing.

Fish Stock

After straining, makes about 2 quarts.
Each 1 cup serving: 3 grams protein • 1 gram carbohydrate

2 pounds fresh fish trimmings
(preferably white fish)

2 large quartered onions

3 celery stalks with leaves,
cut into 2-inch pieces

1 teaspoon grated lemon zest

½ bunch coarsely chopped fresh
parsley

2 bay leaves

2 sprigs fresh thyme, or
1 teaspoon dried thyme

10 whole black peppercorns

2 quarts water

2 cups dry white wine

In a large heavy-bottomed soup pot, bring all ingredients to a boil. Reduce heat to simmer and cook, uncovered, 30 minutes, skimming off any foam that may collect on top.

Strain stock through a fine-meshed sieve. Thoroughly cool before refrigerating or freezing for future use.

Vegetable Stock

After straining, makes about 3 quarts.
Each 1 cup serving: 2 grams protein • 3 grams carbohydrate

2 large quartered onions

2 well-washed, large, coarsely
   chopped leeks

4 carrots, cut into 2-inch pieces

4 celery stalks with leaves, cut
   into 2-inch pieces

2 zucchini, cut into 1-inch
   rounds

2 parsnips, cut into 2-inch
   chunks

4 to 5 fresh thyme sprigs, or
   2 teaspoons dried thyme leaves

6 to 12 whole black peppercorns

1 bunch fresh parsley

4 quarts water

**plus any optional vegetables
on hand, such as:**

½ pound quartered brown or
   white mushrooms

1 chopped bell pepper

any shredded greens, such as
   spinach or Swiss chard

In a large heavy-bottomed stock pot, bring all ingredients to a boil
over high heat. Reduce heat to low and simmer, uncovered, 45 minutes.
Using a fine-meshed sieve, strain stock and discard vegetables. Refrigerate or freeze for future use.

Meat Soups

Charlotte Cady's Ground Beef Soup

Makes 8 servings • Each serving: 20 grams protein • 8 grams carbohydrate

1 pound ground beef

1 cup diced onion

2 garlic cloves

1 diced green bell pepper

8 cups beef stock (see recipe, page 112), or low-sodium canned, or water

2 cups diced carrots

1 cup diced celery stalks

2 cups chopped tomatoes

1 head broccoli, cut into florets, with stalks, peeled and diced

¼ cup minced fresh parsley

1 teaspoon dried thyme

1 teaspoon dried oregano

freshly ground black pepper, to taste

In a large nonstick skillet, sauté ground beef over medium heat, stirring with a wooden spoon to break up lumps. Add onion, garlic and bell pepper and continue sautéing until meat is tender and vegetables have softened, about 5 minutes. Drain fat from pan and set meat mixture aside.

In a large heavy-bottomed soup pot, heat beef stock or water over medium-high heat until boiling. Add carrots and celery and cook until almost tender, about 5 minutes. Add tomatoes, broccoli, parsley, thyme, oregano, black pepper and reserved meat mixture. Mix well. Simmer over low heat 10 minutes, until all vegetables are tender. Taste, and adjust seasonings.

Split Pea Soup with Ham

Makes 6 servings • Each serving: 18 grams protein • 7 grams carbohydrate

1 cup split peas, picked over and rinsed

1 meaty ham bone

8 cups beef stock (see recipe, page 112), or vegetable stock (see recipe, page 115), or low-sodium canned, or water

2 tablespoons pure-pressed extra virgin olive oil

1 medium finely chopped onion

2 minced garlic cloves

2 finely chopped celery stalks with leaves

2 medium diced carrots

2 bay leaves

1 teaspoon ground cumin

freshly ground black pepper, to taste

In a large heavy-bottomed soup pot, bring split peas, ham bone and stock or water to a boil over medium-high heat. Reduce heat to low. Cover and simmer 30 minutes, skimming off any foam that may collect on surface.

In a large nonstick skillet, heat oil over medium-high heat. When oil is hot, add onion, garlic, celery, carrots, bay leaves, cumin and black pepper. Cook until vegetables have softened, about 10 minutes. Add sautéed vegetables to soup pot and simmer, uncovered, 1 hour, or until peas are tender.

Remove ham bone from soup. Shred meat and add to soup. Taste, and adjust seasonings.

Before adding shredded meat, if desired, purée soup in batches in a blender or food processor. Add shredded meat to soup and purée.

Seafood Soups

Classic Bouillabaisse

Makes 8 servings • Each serving: 40 grams protein • 9 grams carbohydrate

3 assorted fresh fish fillets, cut
into 1½-inch chunks
(red snapper, halibut, sea
bass, sole, cod, flounder)

2 dozen small, tightly closed clams

1 dozen tightly closed mussels

½ pound sea scallops

½ pound raw medium shrimp,
peeled and deveined

3 tablespoons pure-pressed extra
virgin olive oil

1 large thinly sliced onion

2 minced garlic cloves

1 cup thinly sliced fresh fennel
bulb

3 large ripe tomatoes, peeled,
seeded and chopped*

1 sprig fresh thyme, or
½ teaspoon dried thyme

1 tablespoon finely chopped fresh
parsley

¼ teaspoon crushed fennel seeds

2 bay leaves

1 teaspoon grated orange zest

2 quarts fish stock (see recipe,
page 114), or clam juice,
diluted by half with water

1 teaspoon crumbled saffron
threads

freshly ground black pepper,
to taste

dash cayenne pepper

8 sprigs fresh parsley, for garnish

Rinse fish under cold water and pat dry with paper towels. Cut into 1½-inch chunks. Scrub clams and mussels. Rinse scallops and shrimp under cold water. Set all seafood aside.

---

*To peel and seed tomatoes: Plunge tomatoes into boiling water for several seconds, then into cold water. The skins will slip off easily. Cut tomatoes in half and squeeze gently. Scoop out seeds using a small spoon or your fingers. Chop tomatoes.

In a large heavy-bottomed soup pot, heat oil over medium-high heat. When oil is hot, add onion and garlic and sauté until softened, about 5 minutes. Add fennel, tomatoes, thyme, parsley, fennel seed, bay leaves and orange zest, and cook over medium heat 5 minutes.

Add fish stock or diluted clam juice. Bring to a boil. Reduce heat to low and simmer, uncovered, 20 minutes. Add saffron threads, black pepper and cayenne pepper. Taste, and adjust seasonings.

Add fish and shellfish in stages: Put in thicker-flesh chunks of fish first and simmer over low heat, covered, 5 minutes. Next add thinner-flesh chunks of fish, clams, mussels, scallops and shrimp. Cover and steam 5 minutes, until shells have opened. Discard any unopened clams or mussels.

Spoon into large soup bowls. Garnish with a sprig of parsley.

Lobster Bisque

Makes 4 servings • Each serving: 16 grams protein • 7 grams carbohydrate

4 tablespoons unsalted butter

1 medium chopped onion

1 minced garlic clove

1 diced carrot

1 finely chopped celery stalk

2 uncooked medium lobster tails, cut into 3 sections each

3½ cups fish stock (see recipe, page 114), or vegetable stock (see recipe, page 115), or low-sodium canned

1 cup dry white wine

1 bay leaf

2 fresh thyme sprigs, or 1 teaspoon dried thyme

2 tablespoons finely chopped fresh parsley

1 tablespoon fresh lemon juice

3 tablespoons unsalted butter

3 tablespoons flour

2 cups all-dairy heavy cream

2 peeled, seeded and coarsely chopped ripe tomatoes,* or 1 tablespoon tomato paste

dash cayenne pepper

1 tablespoon minced fresh chives, for garnish

In a large nonstick skillet, melt butter over medium-high heat. When butter is hot and bubbly, add onion, garlic, carrot and celery, and cook until softened, about 5 minutes.

Add lobster chunks and sauté 2 to 3 minutes. Add fish stock or vegetable stock, wine, bay leaf, thyme, parsley and lemon juice. Reduce heat to low. Cover and simmer 5 to 7 minutes, until lobster shells turn red. Remove lobster from pan and cool. Remove bay leaf. Extract lobster meat from shells, dice into small pieces and set aside.

In a separate saucepan, melt 3 tablespoons butter over medium-high heat. When butter is hot and bubbly, reduce heat to low, sprinkle in flour and blend with a whisk until smooth, about 3 minutes.

---

*To peel and seed tomatoes: Plunge tomatoes into boiling water for several seconds, then into cold water. The skins will slip off easily. Cut tomatoes in half and squeeze gently. Scoop out seeds using a small spoon or your fingers. Chop tomatoes.

In another saucepan, heat cream to almost boiling. *Do not boil.* Add hot cream to flour mixture all at once and whisk constantly over low heat until well blended and thickened, about 2 minutes.

Add 1 cup of hot broth from soup stock to cream sauce and whisk until smooth. Then add all of the cream sauce to broth in soup pot and whisk until well blended.

Stir in tomatoes or tomato paste and cayenne pepper. Simmer gently over low heat 15 minutes, stirring occasionally. Pour soup through a fine-meshed sieve, pressing down on vegetables. Return soup to pot. Add reserved diced lobster. Heat through. *Do not boil.* Taste, and adjust seasonings. Garnish with minced fresh chives.

Salmon Chowder with Pesto Swirl

Makes 4 servings • Each serving: 41 grams protein • 17 grams carbohydrate

3 tablespoons unsalted butter

1 large chopped onion

1 minced garlic clove

1 diced red bell pepper

3 red potatoes (peeled, if desired), diced into ½-inch cubes

4 cups fish stock (see recipe, page 114), or vegetable stock (see recipe, page 115), or low-sodium canned

freshly ground black pepper, to taste

1 pound salmon fillet, skinned, boned, and cut into 1-inch pieces

1 cup all-dairy heavy cream

½ cup Basil Pesto (see recipe, page 372), or store-bought

1 cup fresh green peas or frozen and thawed

4 whole basil leaves, for garnish

In a large heavy-bottomed soup pot, melt butter over medium-high heat. When butter is hot and bubbly, add onion, garlic and bell pepper and sauté until softened, about 5 minutes. Stir in potatoes, stock and black pepper. Bring to a boil, reduce heat to low and simmer until potatoes are tender, about 10 minutes.

Add salmon pieces and cream, and simmer over low heat until salmon flakes easily with a fork, about 5 minutes. Using a fork, swirl in pesto and peas and heat gently. *Do not boil.* Taste, and adjust seasonings. Garnish bowls with whole basil leaves.

Traditional New England Clam Chowder

Makes 4 servings • Each serving: 14 grams protein • 12 grams carbohydrate

2 dozen tightly closed clams, or 18 ounces canned chopped clams (with liquid)

4 cups fish stock (see recipe, page 114), or clam juice diluted by half with water

4 slices nitrate-free bacon

2 tablespoons unsalted butter

1 medium finely chopped onion

1 minced garlic clove

1 finely chopped celery stalk

3 medium red potatoes, (peeled, if desired) diced into ½-inch cubes

1 bay leaf

2 cups all-dairy heavy cream

¼ teaspoon white pepper

2 tablespoons minced fresh chives, for garnish

If using fresh clams, scrub thoroughly, making sure clams are all tightly shut. In a heavy saucepan, bring clams, fish stock or clam juice and water to a boil. Cover and reduce heat to low. Steam until clams open, about 8 to 10 minutes. Discard any clams that did not open. Remove opened clams from shells and coarsely chop. Set aside. Strain broth through a fine-meshed sieve and reserve liquid.

In a nonstick skillet, cook bacon over low heat until crisp. Remove from pan and blot dry on paper towels. Crumble and set aside.

In a heavy-bottomed soup pot, melt butter over medium-high heat. When butter is hot and bubbly, add onion, garlic and celery and sauté until softened, about 5 minutes. Add potatoes and stir until well coated with butter. Add strained stock and bay leaf. Bring to a boil, reduce heat to low and cook, uncovered, until potatoes are tender, about 10 to 15 minutes.

Stir in cream, chopped clams, crumbled bacon and white pepper. Simmer over low heat until heated through, about 5 minutes. *Do not boil.* Taste, and adjust seasonings. Serve garnished with chives sprinkled on top.

Vegetable Soups

Broccoli Potato Cheese Soup

Makes 6 servings • Each serving: 9 grams protein • 11 grams carbohydrate

4 tablespoons unsalted butter

1 well-washed diced leek

1 minced garlic clove

1 diced carrot

3 diced medium red potatoes
(peeled, if desired)

4 cups chicken stock (see recipe,
page 113), or vegetable stock
(see recipe, page 115), or
low-sodium canned

1 bay leaf

½ teaspoon celery seed

2 sprigs fresh thyme, or
1 teaspoon dried thyme

¼ cup slivered fresh basil, or
2 teaspoons dried basil

1 bunch broccoli, cut into
bite-size florets, with stalks
peeled and chopped

1 cup all-dairy heavy cream

freshly ground black pepper,
to taste

dash cayenne pepper

1 cup grated Monterey Jack
cheese

6 whole basil leaves, for garnish

In a large heavy-bottomed soup pot, melt butter over medium-high heat. When butter is hot and bubbly, add leeks, garlic and carrots and cook until softened, about 3 minutes. Add potatoes, stir well and cook 2 minutes.

Add stock, bay leaf, celery seed, thyme and basil. Bring to a boil. Reduce heat to medium and cook until potatoes are barely tender, about 15 minutes. Add broccoli and cook about another 10 minutes, until tender.

In a blender or food processor, purée soup in batches until vegetables are well blended. Pour soup back into pot and stir in cream. Season to taste with black pepper and dash cayenne pepper. Cook over low heat until heated through. *Do not boil.* Stir in cheese just before serving. Taste, and adjust seasonings. Garnish with fresh basil leaves.

Cream of Mushroom Soup

Makes 4 servings • Each serving: 8 grams protein • 5 grams carbohydrate

2 tablespoons unsalted butter

1 cup minced onion

1 minced garlic clove

1 pound thinly sliced brown
   or white mushrooms

1 tablespoon flour

4 cups beef stock (see recipe,
   page 112), chicken stock
   (see recipe, page 113); or
   vegetable stock (see recipe,
   page 115), or low-sodium
   canned

1 tablespoon finely chopped
   fresh parsley

1 bay leaf

¼ teaspoon nutmeg, or
   ½ teaspoon dried thyme

dash cayenne pepper

1 cup all-dairy heavy cream

4 sprigs fresh parsley, for garnish

In a large heavy-bottomed soup pot, melt butter over medium-high heat. When butter is hot and bubbly, add onion and garlic and sauté until softened, about 5 minutes. Add mushrooms and cook until they release their liquid and soften, about 5 more minutes.

Sprinkle flour over onion and mushroom mixture and cook over low heat, stirring, 3 to 4 minutes. Gradually add stock, parsley, bay leaf, nutmeg or thyme and cayenne pepper. Bring to a boil, stirring constantly. Reduce heat and simmer gently 20 minutes, stirring occasionally. Stir in cream. Simmer until heated through. *Do not boil.*

Taste, and adjust seasonings. Garnish bowls with a sprig of fresh parsley.

Creamy Roasted Eggplant Soup

Makes 4 servings • Each serving: 6 grams protein • 17 grams carbohydrate

2 medium eggplants

1 red bell pepper or ¼ cup store-bought roasted red pepper

2 tablespoons unsalted butter

1 medium diced onion

1 minced garlic clove

4 cups vegetable stock (see recipe, page 115), or chicken stock (see recipe, page 113), or low-sodium canned

3 tablespoons Basil or Cilantro Pesto (see recipes, page 372), or store-bought

1 cup all-dairy heavy cream

freshly ground black pepper, to taste

dash cayenne pepper

whole cilantro sprigs, for garnish

Preheat oven to 425°. Cut eggplant in half lengthwise and puncture skin in several places with a fork. Place cut-side down, on a lightly greased baking sheet. Bake until flesh is tender and skin is shriveled and blistered, about 25-35 minutes. Remove from heat and cool. Remove skin from eggplants and discard. Drain pulp in a colander, pressing out as much of the liquid as possible. Coarsely chop eggplant pulp and set aside.

If using a fresh red bell pepper, roast pepper directly over a gas flame or under preheated broiler on a broiler rack. Using tongs, turn pepper frequently, until blistered and blackened on all sides. Place pepper in a bowl with a plate on top. Let steam for 15 minutes to loosen skin. Peel off all charred skin. Dice roasted flesh and set aside.

In a large heavy-bottomed soup pot, melt butter over medium-high heat. When butter is hot and bubbly, add onion and garlic and sauté until softened, about 5 minutes. Add red pepper and eggplant.

Add vegetable or chicken stock and bring to a boil. Reduce heat to low and simmer 20 minutes. In a food processor or blender, purée soup in batches until smooth. Return purée to soup pot and stir in Basil or Cilantro Pesto and cream. Season to taste with black pepper and cayenne pepper. *Do not boil.* Taste, and adjust seasonings. Garnish with whole cilantro sprigs.

Creamy Spinach Soup

Makes 4 servings • Each serving: 7 grams protein • 6 grams carbohydrate

4 bunches spinach equal to about
    4 cups cooked spinach, well
    drained and chopped; or
    32 ounces packaged frozen
    spinach, thawed, drained
    and chopped

4 tablespoons unsalted butter

1 medium diced onion

1 minced garlic clove

1 tablespoon flour

1 teaspoon Dijon mustard

4 cups chicken stock (see recipe,
    page 113), or vegetable stock
    (see recipe, page 115), or
    low-sodium canned

1½ cups all-dairy heavy cream

¼ cup slivered fresh basil, or
    2 teaspoons dried basil

freshly ground black pepper,
    to taste

dash cayenne pepper

whole basil leaves, for garnish

Wash fresh spinach well, removing stems. With water still clinging to leaves, place in a medium saucepan with a tight-fitting lid. Turn heat to medium-high and steam until leaves are wilted, about 2 to 3 minutes. Drain in a colander, pressing out all liquid with the back of a wooden spoon. Chop fine and set aside.

In a heavy-bottomed soup pot, melt butter over medium-high heat. When butter is hot and bubbly, add onion and garlic and sauté until softened, about 5 minutes.

Reduce heat to low, sprinkle in flour and cook 3 to 4 minutes, stirring. *Do not brown.* Stir in mustard and stock. Blend well. Bring to a boil, reduce heat to low and cook, stirring, until slightly thickened and smooth, about 15 minutes. Add cream, chopped spinach, basil, black pepper and cayenne pepper. Mix well.

In a blender or food processor, purée soup in batches until smooth and creamy. Return puréed soup to soup pot and cook over low heat until heated through. *Do not boil.* Taste, and adjust seasonings. Serve garnished with whole basil leaves.

Creamy Tomato Soup

Makes 4 servings • Each serving: 8 grams protein • 20 grams carbohydrate

3 pounds peeled, seeded and
  finely chopped fresh tomatoes*;
  or 28 ounces canned plum
  tomatoes, with juice

1 tablespoon unsalted butter

1 tablespoon pure-pressed extra
  virgin olive oil

1 medium diced onion

2 minced garlic cloves

1 diced carrot

1 diced celery stalk
  with leaves

½ cup sun-dried tomatoes in
  olive oil, drained and chopped

¼ cup finely chopped fresh parsley

⅓ cup slivered fresh basil, or
  2 teaspoons dried basil

1 bay leaf

3 cups chicken stock (see recipe,
  page 113), or vegetable stock
  (see recipe, page 115), or
  low-sodium canned

freshly ground black pepper,
  to taste

1 cup all-dairy heavy cream

In a large heavy-bottomed soup pot, heat butter and oil over medium-high heat. When hot, add onion, garlic, carrots and celery. Sauté until vegetables are softened, about 5 minutes. Add fresh tomatoes and their juice, sun-dried tomatoes, parsley, basil, bay leaf, stock and black pepper. Bring to a boil. Reduce heat to low, partially cover, and simmer 30 minutes, stirring occasionally.

Remove bay leaf. In a blender or food processor, purée soup in batches until smooth. Return soup to pot and stir in cream. Taste and adjust seasonings, and simmer until heated through, about 5 minutes. *Do not boil.*

---

*To peel and seed tomatoes: Plunge tomatoes into boiling water for several seconds, then into cold water. The skins will slip off easily. Cut tomatoes in half and squeeze gently. Scoop out seeds using a small spoon or your fingers. Chop tomatoes.

French Onion Soup

Makes 6 servings • Each serving: 12 grams protein • 3 grams carbohydrate

3 tablespoons unsalted butter

4 large thinly sliced red onions

1 minced garlic clove

6 cups beef stock (see recipe, page 112), or low-sodium canned

½ teaspoon dried thyme

freshly ground black pepper, to taste

1 cup grated Gruyère cheese

¼ cup grated Parmesan cheese

In a heavy-bottomed soup pot, melt butter over medium-high heat. When butter is hot and bubbly, add onion and garlic and sauté over medium-low heat, stirring occasionally, until well softened, about 30 minutes.

Add beef stock, thyme and black pepper. Bring to a boil, reduce heat and simmer, uncovered, over low heat for 30 minutes. Preheat broiler. Divide soup into 6 oven-proof serving bowls. Top with Gruyère and Parmesan cheeses. Place on top rack of oven and broil until cheese is bubbly and melted.

Italian Mixed Vegetable Soup

Makes 6 servings • Each serving: 11 grams protein • 25 grams carbohydrate

2 tablespoons pure-pressed extra virgin olive oil

1 medium finely chopped onion

1 minced garlic clove

1 diced green or red bell pepper

1 chopped celery stalk with leaves

1 diced carrot

1 large diced red potato (peeled, if desired)

¼ pound green beans, ends trimmed, and sliced diagonally into 1-inch pieces

1 medium diced zucchini

28 ounces canned peeled plum tomatoes, chopped (reserve liquid)

4 cups chicken stock (see recipe, page 113), or low-sodium canned

2 bay leaves

1 teaspoon dried oregano

1 teaspoon dried basil

1 teaspoon dried marjoram

freshly ground black pepper, to taste

13¾ ounces canned pinto beans, drained and rinsed

2 tablespoons chopped fresh parsley

2 tablespoons grated Parmesan cheese, for topping

In a large heavy-bottomed soup pot, heat oil over medium-high heat. When oil is hot, add onion, garlic and bell pepper and sauté until softened, about 5 minutes. Add celery, carrot, potato and green beans. Cook, stirring occasionally, 5 minutes. Add zucchini, tomatoes and their liquid, stock, bay leaves, oregano, basil, marjoram and black pepper. Bring to a boil. Reduce heat to low and simmer, covered, until vegetables are tender, about 15 to 20 minutes.

Add pinto beans and parsley and cook until heated through. Taste, and adjust seasonings.

Sprinkle with Parmesan cheese before serving.

Salads

Chicken Salads

Meat Salads

Seafood Salads

Vegetable Salads

Chicken Salads

California Chicken Salad

Makes 4 main-course servings • Each serving: 30 grams protein • 6 grams carbohydrate

~

1 cup raw pecans

1 pound skinless, boneless chicken breasts

2 bay leaves

1 tablespoon pure-pressed extra virgin olive oil

½ thinly sliced red onion

12 spears asparagus, tough ends trimmed, steamed and sliced diagonally into 2-inch pieces

½ cup slivered fresh basil or 2 teaspoons dried basil or 1 tablespoon minced fresh parsley

grated zest of 1 lemon

6 cups mixed salad greens

Put pecans in an ungreased nonstick skillet over medium-high heat. Stir nuts or shake pan almost constantly, until pecans are evenly browned and toasted. Remove from pan immediately and set aside to cool.

Bring 1 inch of water and bay leaves to a boil in a skillet. Reduce heat to medium. Add chicken, cover and poach until cooked through, about 20 minutes, turning once. *Do not overcook.* Let cool and shred with your fingers into julienned strips.

In a small skillet, heat oil over medium-high heat. When oil is hot, add onion and sauté until softened, about 5 minutes.

In a large bowl combine sautéed onions with chicken, asparagus pieces, basil or parsley and lemon zest. Toss with Balsamic Vinaigrette.

Line 4 individual plates with washed and dried salad greens. Spoon chicken salad over greens. Sprinkle roasted pecans over the top.

Balsamic Dressing

1 tablespoon Dijon mustard

1 minced garlic clove

½ cup balsamic vinegar

½ cup pure-pressed extra virgin olive oil

freshly ground black pepper, to taste

In a small bowl, using a fork, whisk all of the ingredients until well blended and smooth. Taste, and adjust seasonings.

Chinese Chicken Salad

Makes 4 main-course servings • Each serving: 33 grams protein • 3 grams carbohydrate

4 boneless, skinless chicken breasts

2 bay leaves

1 medium jicama, peeled and sliced into matchstick pieces; or 12 sliced water chestnuts, rinsed and drained

Chinese Chicken Salad Dressing

6 cups mixed salad greens

½ cup dry-roasted peanuts

3 minced celery stalks, sliced into thin sticks then cut diagonally into 1-inch length strips

3 minced scallions

1 red bell pepper, cut into thin strips

1 tablespoon minced fresh cilantro

Bring 1 inch of water and bay leaves to a boil in a skillet. Reduce heat to medium. Add chicken, cover and poach until cooked through, about 20 minutes, turning once. *Do not overcook.* Let cool and julienne into bite-sized strips.

In a large bowl, combine chicken, jicama or water chestnuts, celery, scallions and bell pepper. Mix with Chinese Chicken Salad Dressing.

Line 4 individual plates with washed and dried salad greens. Arrange chicken salad over greens. Sprinkle with peanuts and cilantro.

Chinese Chicken Salad Dressing

1 teaspoon peeled and finely minced fresh ginger

2 minced garlic cloves

1 tablespoon low-sodium tamari soy sauce

2 tablespoons fresh lime juice

¼ cup pure-pressed sesame oil

½ cup mayonnaise (made from pure-pressed oil)

In a blender or food processor, blend all ingredients until smooth, or place ingredients in a jar with a tight-fitting lid and shake vigorously until well blended. Taste, and adjust seasonings.

Classic Chicken Salad

Makes 4 main-course servings • Each serving: 29 grams protein • 3 grams carbohydrate

2 bay leaves

4 boneless, skinless chicken breasts

2 teaspoons minced fresh parsley

½ cup finely diced celery stalks

½ cup chopped raw pecans

⅔ cup mayonnaise (made from
  pure-pressed oil)

2 teaspoons Dijon mustard

1 teaspoon curry powder
  (optional)

freshly ground black pepper,
  to taste

6 cups mixed salad greens

Creamy Vinaigrette

4 fresh parsley sprigs, for garnish

Bring 1 inch of water and bay leaves to a boil in a skillet. Reduce heat to medium. Add chicken, cover, and poach until cooked through, about 20 minutes, turning once. *Do not overcook.* Let cool and shred with fingers.

In a large bowl, combine all ingredients except salad greens, vinaigrette and parsley sprigs. Blend well with a fork. Taste, and adjust seasonings.

Line 4 individual plates with washed and dried salad greens. Mound greens with chicken salad and garnish with whole parsley sprigs. Pass Creamy Vinaigrette on the side.

Creamy Vinaigrette

½ cup red wine vinegar

2 teaspoons Dijon mustard

2 tablespoons fresh lemon juice

1 minced garlic clove

1 to 2 teaspoons peeled and finely
  minced fresh ginger (optional)

1 cup pure-pressed extra virgin
  olive oil

freshly ground black pepper,
  to taste

In a blender or food processor, combine all ingredients and blend until smooth; or place ingredients in a jar with a tight-fitting lid, and shake vigorously until well blended. Taste, and adjust seasonings.

Mexican Chicken Salad

Makes 4 main-course servings • Each serving: 31 grams protein • 9 grams carbohydrate

4 boneless, skinless chicken breasts

1 cup fresh steamed corn
(or frozen and thawed)

3 seeded and diced tomatoes*

2 tablespoons minced fresh
cilantro

1 small minced fresh jalapeño
pepper; or 1 to 2 tablespoons
canned diced green chilies,
to taste [wear rubber gloves to
prepare fresh jalapeño pepper]

1 diced red bell pepper

¼ cup diced red onion

¼ cup chopped scallions

½ cup sliced black or green olives

6 cups fresh spinach, washed,
stemmed and torn into
bite-size pieces

Mexican Chicken Salad Dressing
(see recipe, page 137)

4 sprigs fresh cilantro, for garnish

In a medium, covered skillet, poach chicken in 1 inch of water with 2
bay leaves over medium heat until cooked through, about 20 minutes.
Do not overcook. Let cool and shred with fingers.

In a large bowl, combine all ingredients except spinach and cilantro
sprigs. Mix with salad dressing. Line 4 individual plates with washed
and dried spinach leaves. Top with a scoop of chicken salad. Garnish
with a sprig of fresh cilantro.

———————

*To seed tomatoes: Cut tomatoes in half and squeeze gently. Scoop out seeds using a small spoon
or your fingers. Dice tomatoes.

Mexican Chicken Salad Dressing

¼ cup fresh lime juice

1 teaspoon dried oregano

1 teaspoon ground cumin

2 minced garlic cloves

½ cup mayonnaise (made from
  pure-pressed oil)

¼ cup pure-pressed vegetable oil

freshly ground black pepper,
  to taste

In a blender or food processor, blend all ingredients until smooth, or place ingredients in a jar with a tight-fitting lid and shake vigorously until well blended. Taste, and adjust seasonings.

Santa Barbara Cobb Salad

Makes 4 main-course servings • Each serving: 35 grams protein • 6 grams carbohydrate

4 diced hard-boiled eggs	*1 cup crumbled bleu cheese*
2 bay leaves	*2 medium chopped tomatoes*
2 boneless, skinless chicken breasts	*1 large, diced, ripe avocado*
8 slices nitrate-free bacon, cooked and crumbled	*6 chopped scallions*
	6 cups mixed salad greens
	Cobb Dressing

To hard boil eggs, place eggs in a saucepan and cover with cold water. Bring to a boil uncovered. Allow to boil for 1 minute then cover, remove from heat and let sit undisturbed 10 minutes. Rinse eggs under cold water. Crack shells, peel and rinse eggs.

Bring 1 inch of water and bay leaves to a boil in a skillet. Reduce heat to medium. Add chicken, cover and poach until cooked through, about 20 minutes, turning once. *Do not overcook.* Let cool and dice.

In a large bowl, mix all ingredients except salad greens and dressing. Arrange salad greens on 4 individual chilled plates. Mix chicken mixture with some of the Cobb Dressing, and mound on top of greens. Pass remaining dressing on the side.

Cobb Dressing

1 tablespoon Dijon mustard	*freshly ground black pepper, to taste*
1 minced garlic clove	
2 tablespoons fresh lemon juice	*½ cup pure-pressed extra virgin olive oil*
1 tablespoon red wine vinegar	

In a small bowl, using a fork, whisk mustard, garlic, lemon juice, vinegar and pepper. Drizzle oil in a steady stream while continuing to whisk, until dressing is thickened and creamy. Taste, and adjust seasonings.

Meat Salads

Antipasto Plate

Makes 4 main-course servings • Each serving: 42 grams protein • 18 grams carbohydrate

1 head washed and dried butter
lettuce

⅓ cup green olives

⅓ cup Kalamata olives

1 small thinly sliced red onion

1 cup marinated mushrooms

1 cup roasted red bell peppers

1 cup marinated artichoke hearts

1 cup garbanzo beans in
vinaigrette

2 large ripe tomatoes, sliced into
eighths

⅓ cup hot Greek peppers

½ pound thinly sliced nitrate-
free ham

½ pound thinly sliced mozzarella
cheese

Antipasto Dressing

Place salad leaves on a large platter. Arrange all antipasto ingredi
ents on top of lettuce in a decorative manner. Pass Antipasto Dressing
on the side.

Antipasto Dressing

2 tablespoons balsamic vinegar

1 tablespoon red wine vinegar

½ cup pure-pressed extra virgin
olive oil

1 minced garlic clove

1 teaspoon dried oregano

freshly ground black pepper,
to taste

In a small bowl, using a fork, whisk all of the ingredients until well
blended and smooth. Taste, and adjust seasonings.

Classic Chef's Salad

Makes 4 main-course servings.
Each serving (not including dressing): 40 grams protein • 3 grams carbohydrate

2 boneless, skinless chicken breasts

2 bay leaves

6 cups mixed salad greens

8 ounces cooked, cold, nitrate-free
ham, cut into thin strips

8 ounces Swiss cheese, cut into
thin strips

2 medium-ripe quartered
tomatoes

2 hard-boiled eggs, quartered*

1 cup sliced brown or white
mushrooms

1 cup thinly sliced celery

1 cup peeled and sliced cucumber

1 cup pitted black Greek or green
olives

your choice of dressing (see
Salad Dressings, starting on
page 179)

Bring 1 inch of water and bay leaves to a boil in a skillet. Reduce heat
to medium, add chicken, cover and poach until cooked through, about 20
minutes, turning once. *Do not overcook.* Let cool and dice.

Tear salad greens into bite-size pieces and put in a large salad bowl.
Arrange remaining ingredients on top of salad. Toss with dressing, or
pass dressing on the side. Serve on chilled salad plates.

---

*To hard boil eggs, place eggs in a medium saucepan and cover with cold water. Bring to a boil
uncovered. Allow to boil for 1 minute, then cover, remove from heat and let sit undisturbed for 10
minutes. Rinse eggs under cold water. Crack shells, peel and rinse eggs.

Spinach Salad with Bacon, Avocado and Mushrooms

Makes 4 side-dish servings • Each serving: 8 grams protein • 8 grams carbohydrate

1 pound fresh spinach leaves, washed, dried and torn into bite-size pieces

8 slices nitrate-free bacon, cooked and crumbled

2 ripe avocados, peeled, diced and sprinkled with fresh lemon juice

8 ounces thinly sliced brown or white mushrooms

¼ cup diced scallions

Garlic Dijon Vinaigrette

Place spinach in a large serving bowl. Arrange bacon, avocado, mushrooms and scallions over top. Toss with Garlic Dijon Vinaigrette and serve immediately.

Garlic Dijon Vinaigrette

3 tablespoons balsamic vinegar

2 minced garlic cloves

1 tablespoon Dijon mustard

1 tablespoon slivered fresh basil, or 1 teaspoon dried basil

¾ cup pure-pressed extra virgin olive oil

freshly ground black pepper, to taste

Combine all ingredients in a jar with a tight-fitting lid and shake vigorously until well blended and smooth. Taste, and adjust seasonings.

Steak Salad

Makes 4 main-dish servings • Each serving: 28 grams protein • 2 grams carbohydrate

4 cups mixed salad greens	½ small thinly sliced red onion
1 pound lean sirloin steak, grilled or broiled, trimmed of fat and thinly sliced	Salsa Dressing

Line 4 individual plates with salad greens. Arrange steak slices on top of salad. Sprinkle with onion slices and top with Salsa Dressing.

Salsa Dressing

2 large seeded and diced tomatoes*	2 tablespoons minced red onion
1 minced garlic clove	2 tablespoons finely chopped fresh cilantro
1 small minced fresh jalapeño pepper; or 1 to 2 tablespoons canned diced green chilies to taste [wear rubber gloves to prepare fresh jalapeño pepper]	1 teaspoon fresh lime juice
	1 tablespoon pure-pressed extra virgin olive oil
	freshly ground black pepper, to taste

In a medium bowl, using a fork, combine all ingredients. Taste, and adjust seasonings.

---

*To seed tomatoes: Cut tomatoes in half and squeeze gently. Scoop out seeds using a small spoon or your fingers. Dice tomatoes.

Seafood Salads

Salade Niçoise

Makes 4 main-dish servings • Each serving: 30 grams protein • 7 grams carbohydrate

16 green beans, ends trimmed

2 large red potatoes (peeled, if desired)

French Vinaigrette (see recipe, page 144)

1 head butter or romaine lettuce, washed, with leaves torn into large pieces

2 hard-boiled eggs, sliced into quarters lengthwise*

½ cup Greek, Niçoise green or black olives

1 tablespoon drained and rinsed capers

13 ounces canned tuna, drained and flaked

2 medium quartered tomatoes

1 ounce canned, drained flat anchovy fillets (optional)

1 tablespoon slivered fresh basil or fresh parsley

1 tablespoon minced scallions

Cook green beans in boiling water until just barely tender, about 5 minutes. Remove with a slotted spoon and rinse under cold water. Drain again and slice diagonally into 1-inch sections.

Cook potatoes in the same boiling water until tender, about 15 to 20 minutes. Cut into 1-inch cubes. Drizzle potatoes with a little French Vinaigrette while still warm. Set aside.

Line a large platter with lettuce leaves. Arrange green beans, potatoes, hard boiled eggs, olives, capers, tuna, tomatoes and anchovies on the lettuce. Sprinkle with fresh basil or parsley and minced scallions.

Spoon French Vinaigrette over salad, or pass dressing on the side. Serve immediately.

---

*To hard boil eggs, place eggs in a medium saucepan and cover with cold water. Bring to a boil uncovered. Allow to boil for 1 minute, then cover, remove from heat and let sit undisturbed 10 minutes. Rinse eggs under cold water. Crack shells, peel and rinse eggs.

French Vinaigrette

⅓ cup red wine vinegar

1½ tablespoons Dijon mustard

⅓ cup pure-pressed extra virgin
   olive oil

1 tablespoon chopped fresh
   parsley

freshly ground black pepper,
   to taste

In a small bowl, using a fork, whisk red wine vinegar and mustard. Slowly drizzle in olive oil, whisking constantly until vinaigrette thickens. Stir in parsley and black pepper and whisk thoroughly. Taste, and adjust seasonings.

Seafood Salad

Makes 4 main-dish servings • Each serving: 45 grams protein • 7 grams carbohydrate

8 ounces shrimp, peeled,
   deveined and cooked

8 ounces flaked crabmeat

8 ounces lightly sautéed scallops

4 minced celery stalks

1 cup fresh green peas, steamed
   until tender and drained,
   or frozen and thawed

6 cups mixed salad greens

1 diced red bell pepper

1 tablespoon minced fresh parsley

1 tablespoon minced scallions

Creamy Curried Dressing

In a large bowl, combine all ingredients except salad greens and dressing. Arrange greens on 4 individual plates. Top with seafood and vegetables. Spoon Creamy Curried Dressing over salad and serve immediately.

Creamy Curried Dressing

½ cup whole sour cream

⅓ cup mayonnaise (made with
   pure-pressed oil)

1 teaspoon curry powder

1 tablespoon fresh lime juice

1 teaspoon grated lime zest

2 teaspoons minced fresh cilantro

1 teaspoon peeled and finely
   minced fresh ginger

freshly ground black pepper,
   to taste

dash cayenne pepper

In a small bowl, using a fork, combine all ingredients until well blended and smooth. Taste, and adjust seasonings.

Seared Salmon or Tuna Salad

Makes 4 side-dish servings • Each serving: 30 grams protein • 4 grams carbohydrate

2 tablespoons pure-pressed extra
  virgin olive oil

1 pound fresh salmon or tuna,
  cut into 4 pieces

1 tablespoon peeled and finely
  minced fresh ginger

2 minced garlic cloves

¼ cup pure-pressed extra virgin
  olive oil

2 tablespoons rice wine vinegar

1 teaspoon fresh lime juice

2 teaspoons drained and rinsed
  capers

freshly ground black pepper,
  to taste

4 cups fresh spinach, washed,
  stemmed and torn into
  bite-size pieces

1 diced ripe avocado

1 tablespoon minced fresh
  cilantro, for garnish

In a large nonstick skillet, heat oil over medium-high heat. When oil is hot, add salmon or tuna and cook quickly, about 15 seconds on each side. Remove from pan. Cut into thin diagonal slices. Set aside.

In a medium bowl, using a fork, mix ginger, garlic, oil, vinegar, lime juice, capers and black pepper. Taste, and adjust seasonings. Pour a little over the seared fish.

Just before serving, toss spinach with some of the dressing. Place spinach leaves on 4 individual plates. Arrange fish and avocado slices on top. Sprinkle with minced cilantro.

Shrimp Salad

Makes 4 side-dish servings • Each serving: 42 grams protein • trace carbohydrate

1 head romaine lettuce (leaves
  left whole), washed and dried

1½ pounds cooked shrimp,
  peeled and deveined

½ cup minced celery stalks

2 tablespoons drained and rinsed
  capers

¼ cup minced scallions

1 tablespoon minced fresh
  cilantro, or parsley

Creamy Vinaigrette

Arrange 3 whole romaine leaves on each of 4 salad plates. Divide shrimp onto leaves. Sprinkle with celery, capers, scallions and cilantro or parsley. Spoon Creamy Vinaigrette over salad.

Creamy Vinaigrette

½ cup red wine vinegar

2 tablespoons Dijon mustard

2 tablespoons fresh lemon juice

1 minced garlic clove

1 teaspoon peeled and finely
  minced fresh ginger

1 cup pure-pressed extra virgin
  olive oil

freshly ground black pepper,
  to taste

Combine all ingredients in a jar with a tight-fitting lid and shake vigorously until well blended. Taste, and adjust seasonings.

Thai Shrimp Salad

Makes 4 side-dish servings • Each serving: 30 grams protein • 4 grams carbohydrate

1 pound cooked shrimp, peeled and deveined

1 cup shredded green cabbage

1 cup steamed sugar peas

4 cups fresh spinach, washed, stemmed and torn into bite-size pieces

1 cup thinly sliced brown or white mushrooms

1 diced red bell pepper

3 finely chopped scallions
Thai Vinaigrette

1 tablespoon minced fresh cilantro, for garnish

½ cup dry-roasted peanuts, for garnish

In a medium bowl, combine shrimp, cabbage, sugar peas, mushrooms, bell pepper and scallions. Toss with half of the Thai Vinaigrette.

Line 4 plates with spinach leaves. Mound shrimp and vegetables on top. Sprinkle with cilantro and peanuts. Serve remaining dressing on the side.

Thai Vinaigrette

2 tablespoons fresh lime juice

2 tablespoons rice wine vinegar

1 tablespoon low-sodium tamari soy sauce

1 minced garlic clove

2 tablespoons minced fresh mint

2 tablespoons slivered fresh basil

2 tablespoons minced fresh cilantro

2 teaspoons peeled and finely minced fresh ginger

1 tablespoon hot chili oil

¼ cup pure-pressed extra virgin olive oil

¼ teaspoon red-pepper flakes (optional)

In a blender or food processor, blend all ingredients until smooth, *or* place ingredients in a jar with a tight-fitting lid and shake vigorously until well blended. Taste, and adjust seasonings.

Tuna or Crab Salad

Makes 4 side-dish servings • Each serving: 23 grams protein • trace carbohydrate

13 ounces canned tuna or crab,
drained and flaked

⅓ cup mayonnaise (made from
pure-pressed oil)

2 teaspoons drained and rinsed
capers

6 cups mixed salad greens

½ cup minced celery stalks

2 tablespoons minced red onion

¼ cup fresh lemon juice

1 tablespoon Dijon mustard

freshly ground black pepper,
to taste

Creamy Vinaigrette

In a medium bowl, using a fork, combine all ingredients, except salad greens and vinaigrette. Mix well.

Line 4 individual plates with salad greens. Scoop tuna or crab salad over mixed greens. Spoon Creamy Vinaigrette over salad.

Creamy Vinaigrette

½ cup red wine vinegar

2 tablespoons Dijon mustard

2 tablespoons fresh lemon juice

1 minced garlic clove

1 cup pure-pressed extra virgin
olive oil

freshly ground black pepper,
to taste

Combine all ingredients in a jar with a tight-fitting lid and shake vigorously until well blended. Taste, and adjust seasonings.

Vegetable Salads

Beet and Onion Salad

Makes 4 side-dish servings • Each serving: 2 grams protein • 11 grams carbohydrate

1 pound fresh steamed, peeled
and julienned beets

1 medium thinly sliced red onion

3 tablespoons slivered fresh basil,
or 3 tablespoons minced fresh
parsley

Beet Vinaigrette

Combine beets, onion and fresh basil or parsley. Pour Beet Vinaigrette over salad and refrigerate 30 minutes before serving.

Beet Vinaigrette

1 tablespoon balsamic vinegar

1 tablespoon red wine vinegar

3 tablespoons pure-pressed extra
virgin olive oil

freshly ground black pepper,
to taste

In a small bowl, using a fork, whisk vinegars, oil and black pepper until smooth.

California Coleslaw

Makes 4 side-dish servings • Each serving: trace protein • trace carbohydrate

1 ½ cups shredded green
cabbage

1 ½ cups shredded red cabbage

1 coarsely grated carrot

3 celery stalks, sliced thin
diagonally

½ thinly sliced red onion
(optional)

¼ cup minced fresh parsley

California Coleslaw Dressing

In a large bowl, toss all ingredients with California Coleslaw Dressing.
Refrigerate at least 1 hour before serving.

California Coleslaw Dressing

½ cup mayonnaise (made from
pure-pressed oil)

¼ cup red wine vinegar

½ teaspoon celery seed

1 teaspoon Dijon mustard

2 tablespoons minced fresh
parsley

freshly ground black pepper,
to taste

In a blender or food processor, blend all ingredients until smooth;
or place ingredients in a jar with a tight-fitting lid and shake vigorously until well blended. Taste, and adjust seasonings.

Caponata Salad

Makes 6 side-dish servings • Each serving: 4 grams protein • 4 grams carbohydrate

2 tablespoons raw pine nuts,
 for garnish

¼ cup pure-pressed extra virgin
 olive oil

1 medium eggplant, cut into
 ½-inch cubes (peeled, if desired)

2 tablespoons pure-pressed extra
 virgin olive oil

3 minced garlic cloves

1 medium chopped red onion

3 chopped celery stalks

1 chopped red bell pepper

one 14-ounce can plum tomatoes,
 drained and chopped (reserve
 liquid)

2 tablespoons drained and rinsed
 capers

½ cup pitted and chopped green
 olives

1 tablespoon chopped fresh
 parsley

1 bay leaf

1 tablespoon balsamic vinegar

½ teaspoon dried oregano

½ teaspoon dried basil

freshly ground black pepper,
 to taste

Put pine nuts in an ungreased skillet over medium-high heat. Stir nuts or shake pan almost constantly, until pine nuts are evenly browned and toasted. Remove from pan immediately and set aside.

In a large nonstick skillet, heat ¼ cup oil over medium-high heat. When oil is hot, add eggplant and sauté until softened and lightly browned, about 10 minutes. Remove from skillet and set aside.

In the same skillet, heat remaining 2 tablespoons oil over medium-high heat. When oil is hot, add garlic, onion, celery and bell pepper, and sauté until softened, about 8 minutes. Add chopped tomatoes, cooked eggplant, capers, olives, bay leaf, parsley, vinegar, oregano, basil and black pepper. Simmer over low heat 20 to 30 minutes, stirring occasionally. Add reserved tomato liquid, if needed, to prevent sticking. Taste, and adjust seasonings.

Spoon into a serving bowl and garnish with toasted pine nuts. Serve at room temperature.

Carrot Salad

Makes 8 side-dish servings • Each serving: 1 gram protein • 1 gram carbohydrate

1 pound shredded carrots

1 fennel bulb (stalk and core
removed), cut into thin strips,
lengthwise

½ cup diced raw walnuts

½ cup chopped fresh parsley

Carrot Salad Dressing

Combine carrots, fennel, walnuts and parsley. Toss with Carrot Salad Dressing and marinate in refrigerator 1 hour before serving.

Carrot Salad Dressing

3 tablespoons fresh lime juice

1 teaspoon ground cumin

freshly ground black pepper,
to taste

2 tablespoons pure-pressed extra
virgin olive oil

In a small bowl, using a fork, whisk lime juice, cumin and black pepper. Slowly drizzle in olive oil, whisking until smooth. Taste, and adjust seasonings.

Classic Egg Salad

Makes 4 servings • Each serving: 16 grams protein • trace carbohydrate

8 hard-boiled eggs

1 tablespoon Dijon mustard

½ cup mayonnaise (made from pure-pressed oil)

1 tablespoon capers, rinsed and drained, (optional)

1 tablespoon minced fresh parsley

½ teaspoon dried dill

freshly ground black pepper, to taste

dash cayenne pepper

To hard boil eggs, place eggs in a saucepan and cover with cold water. Bring to boil uncovered. Allow to boil for one minute, then cover, remove from heat, and let sit undisturbed for 10 minutes. Rinse eggs under cold water. Crack shells, peel and rinse eggs and chop fine.

In a medium bowl combine chopped egg with remaining ingredients. Taste, and adjust seasonings.

Classic Tomato and Mozzarella Salad

Makes 4 side-dish servings • Each serving: 9 grams protein • 6 grams carbohydrate

4 firm, large, very ripe tomatoes
½ pound sliced fresh Buffalo
* mozzarella cheese*

¼ cup slivered fresh basil, or
2 teaspoons dried basil
Classic Vinaigrette

Thinly slice tomatoes and arrange on plates, alternating with mozzarella slices. Sprinkle with fresh basil. Spoon Classic Vinaigrette over salad. Refrigerate 1 hour before serving.

Classic Vinaigrette

2 tablespoons red wine vinegar
3 tablespoons pure-pressed extra
* virgin olive oil*

freshly ground black pepper,
* to taste*

In a small bowl, using a fork, whisk all ingredients until well blended.

Cottage Cheese Salad with Chopped Vegetables

Makes 4 side-dish servings • Each serving: 15 grams protein • 3 grams carbohydrate

2 finely diced carrots

3 finely chopped scallions

1 finely chopped red bell pepper

3 finely chopped celery stalks

1 tablespoon minced fresh parsley

4 cups mixed salad greens

1 tablespoon minced fresh chives

2 cups whole cottage cheese

freshly ground black pepper, to taste

In a medium bowl, using a fork, mix all ingredients, except salad greens, with cottage cheese. Line 4 individual plates with mixed salad greens. Mound cottage cheese salad on top. Serve immediately.

Creamy Marinated Cucumbers

Makes 4 side-dish servings • Each serving: 3 grams protein • 2 grams carbohydrate

3 medium cucumbers, regular
   or hothouse

½ teaspoon salt

Creamy Cucumber Marinade

If using regular waxed cucumbers, peel, cut in half lengthwise, remove seeds and slice into thin half-circles. If using unwaxed hothouse cucumbers, score flesh by running the tines of a fork down sides, making deep incisions. Slice into thin circles. Sprinkle cucumber slices with salt and toss well to coat. Let cucumber drain about 30 minutes in a colander. Rinse well under cold water to remove salt and pat dry with paper towels. Toss with Creamy Cucumber Marinade and marinate 30 minutes before serving.

Creamy Cucumber Marinade

⅔ cup whole sour cream

2 teaspoons minced fresh mint

2 teaspoons minced fresh parsley

2 teaspoons minced scallions

1 minced garlic clove

2 tablespoons fresh lemon juice

freshly ground black pepper,
   to taste

In a medium bowl, using a fork, whisk dressing ingredients. Toss with drained cucumbers. Taste, and adjust seasonings.

Curried Spinach Salad with Almond Dressing

Makes 4 side-dish servings • Each serving: 8 grams protein • 19 grams carbohydrate

1 diced carrot	2 diced celery stalks
1 diced green apple	⅓ cup raisins
6 cups washed and dried spinach leaves	Curried Almond Dressing

In a large bowl, combine carrot, apple, celery and raisins. Arrange spinach leaves on 4 individual salad plates. Mound salad on top of spinach. Pass Curried Almond Dressing on the side.

Curried Almond Dressing

½ cup coarsely chopped raw almonds	1 tablespoon sesame tahini
⅔ cup pure-pressed extra virgin olive oil	1 minced garlic clove
	¼ cup mayonnaise (made from pure-pressed oil)
½ cup fresh lime juice	½ teaspoon curry powder
2 tablespoons fresh orange juice	freshly ground black pepper,
2 teaspoons low-sodium tamari soy sauce	to taste

Put almonds in an ungreased skillet over medium-high heat. Stir or shake pan almost constantly, until almonds are evenly browned and toasted. Remove from pan immediately and set aside.

In a blender or food processor, combine all ingredients with ¼ cup almonds and blend until smooth; or place ingredients in a jar with a tight-fitting lid and shake vigorously until well blended. Stir in remaining almonds. Taste, and adjust seasonings.

Garbanzo Bean Salad

Makes 4 side-dish servings • Each serving: 3 grams protein • 8 grams carbohydrate

13¾ ounces canned garbanzo
beans, drained and rinsed

½ cup chopped red onion

1 cup diced celery stalks

1 cup diced carrot

½ cup minced fresh parsley

1 cup seeded and diced cucumber

1 cup diced red bell pepper

Garbanzo Vinaigrette

In a large bowl, toss all ingredients with Garbanzo Vinaigrette. Cover, and chill 1 hour before serving

Garbanzo Vinaigrette

1 minced garlic clove

2 tablespoons fresh lemon juice

2 tablespoons balsamic vinegar

1 tablespoon Dijon mustard

4 tablespoons pure-pressed extra
virgin olive oil

freshly ground black pepper,
to taste

In a blender or food processor, combine all ingredients and blend until smooth; or place ingredients in a jar with a tight-fitting lid and shake vigorously until well blended. Taste, and adjust seasonings.

Greek Salad

Makes 4 side-dish servings • Each serving: 12 grams protein • 3 grams carbohydrate

1 head romaine lettuce, washed, dried and torn into bite-size pieces

2 tomatoes, cut into chunks

2 cups green beans, ends trimmed, sliced into 1-inch pieces and steamed until just tender

12 Kalamata or any style Greek olives

1 peeled and sliced cucumber

½ thinly sliced red onion

1 cup crumbled feta cheese

2 tablespoons minced fresh parsley, for garnish

Greek Dressing

Line a platter with washed and dried lettuce. Arrange remaining ingredients, except parsley, on top of lettuce. Toss lightly with Greek Dressing. Sprinkle with parsley.

Greek Dressing

2 tablespoons red wine vinegar

1 minced garlic clove

1 tablespoon fresh lemon juice

1 teaspoon Dijon mustard

1 teaspoon dried oregano

½ cup pure-pressed extra virgin olive oil

freshly ground black pepper, to taste

In a blender or food processor, combine all ingredients and blend until smooth; or place ingredients in a jar with a tight-fitting lid and shake vigorously until well blended. Taste, and adjust seasonings.

Green Bean, Feta Cheese and Kalamata Olive Salad

Makes 4 side-dish servings • Each serving: 9 grams protein • 2 grams carbohydrate

1 pound fresh green beans, ends
  trimmed, sliced diagonally
  into 1-inch pieces and steamed
  until tender

½ thinly sliced red onion

⅔ cup pitted and diced
  Kalamata olives

⅔ cup crumbled feta cheese

¼ cup slivered fresh basil, or
  2 teaspoons dried basil

Dijon Garlic Marinade

Combine all ingredients and mix with Dijon Garlic Marinade.

Dijon Garlic Marinade

3 tablespoons balsamic vinegar

1 tablespoon Dijon mustard

2 minced garlic cloves

freshly ground black pepper,
  to taste

3 tablespoons pure-pressed extra
  virgin olive oil

In a small bowl, using a fork, combine vinegar, garlic and black pepper. Slowly drizzle in olive oil, whisking until smooth and well blended. Taste, and adjust seasonings.

Guacamole Salad

Makes 4 side-dish servings • Each serving: 4 grams protein • 9 grams carbohydrate

2 ripe avocados

1 tablespoon fresh lemon juice

*1 seeded and chopped large,
ripe tomato*

1 minced garlic clove

1 tablespoon chopped red onion

*1 tablespoon chopped fresh
cilantro*

*1 small minced fresh jalapeño
pepper (optional),* or *1 to 2
tablespoons canned diced green
chilies, to taste* [wear rubber
gloves to prepare fresh
jalapeño pepper]

*freshly ground black pepper,
to taste*

dash hot-pepper sauce

4 cups mixed salad greens

Cut avocados in half. Remove pits and scoop flesh into a medium bowl. Using a fork, mash avocado with lemon juice.

To seed tomato, cut tomato in half and squeeze gently. Scoop out seeds with a small spoon or your fingers and chop tomato. To mashed avocados, gently mix in tomato, garlic, onion, cilantro, jalapeño pepper, black pepper and hot-pepper sauce. Taste, and adjust seasonings. Serve on a bed of mixed salad greens.

Mixed-Greens Salad

Makes 4 side-dish servings • Each serving: 4 grams protein • 4 grams carbohydrate

4 cups mixed salad greens

Optional Additions

½ cup diced cucumbers

½ cup sliced radishes

1 cup shredded red cabbage

1 cup shredded radicchio

½ cup diced celery stalks

*1 cup sliced brown or white
mushrooms*

½ cup grated carrots

*1 cup thinly sliced red or green
bell peppers*

½ cup thinly sliced fennel

½ cup diced scallions

½ cup thinly sliced red onion

¼ cup raw sunflower seeds

¼ cup diced raw walnuts

In a large bowl, toss ingredients with your choice of dressing. (See Salad Dressings, starting on page 179).

Mixed-Greens Salad with Chèvre (Goat Cheese)

Makes 4 side-dish servings • Each serving: 7 grams protein • trace carbohydrate

four ¾-inch rounds of chèvre (goat cheese) cut from a log of chèvre

¼ cup pure-pressed extra virgin olive oil

2 teaspoons mixed dried Italian herbs (oregano, basil, marjoram, thyme)

4 cups mixed salad greens

Classic Salad Dressing

Place goat cheese rounds in a shallow baking dish. Combine olive oil and herbs and pour over cheese. Marinate several hours or overnight, covered, in refrigerator.

Preheat oven to 375°. Bake cheese 15 minutes or until softened.

Wash and dry greens. Arrange salad greens on individual plates. Place a round of baked goat cheese in center of each plate. Drizzle Classic Salad Dressing over salad greens and serve immediately.

Classic Salad Dressing

½ cup balsamic vinegar

½ cup pure-pressed extra virgin olive oil

freshly ground black pepper, to taste

In a small bowl, using a fork, whisk vinegar, olive oil and black pepper until smooth.

Mixed-Greens Salad with Toasted Walnuts and Gorgonzola Cheese

Makes 4 side-dish servings • Each serving: 9 grams protein • 3 grams carbohydrate

½ cup chopped raw walnuts

4 cups mixed salad greens

Dijon Vinaigrette

½ cup crumbled Gorgonzola
cheese

Put walnuts in an ungreased skillet over medium-high heat. Stir nuts or shake pan almost constantly until walnuts are evenly browned and toasted. Remove from pan immediately and set aside.

In a large bowl, toss salad greens with Dijon Vinaigrette. Sprinkle with toasted walnuts and Gorgonzola cheese.

Dijon Vinaigrette

1 minced garlic clove

2 tablespoons Dijon mustard

¼ cup balsamic vinegar

½ cup pure-pressed extra virgin
olive oil

freshly ground black pepper,
to taste

In a blender or food processor, combine all ingredients and blend until smooth; or place ingredients in a jar with a tight-fitting lid and shake vigorously until well blended. Taste, and adjust seasonings.

Mushroom and Artichoke Salad

Makes 4 side-dish servings • Each serving: 3 grams protein • 7 grams carbohydrate

*1 pound brown or white
 mushrooms, stems removed
 and thickly sliced*
*1 cup marinated artichoke
 hearts, drained and quartered*

4 chopped celery stalks
¼ cup chopped fresh parsley
½ thinly sliced red onion
Mushroom Marinade

Combine mushrooms, artichoke hearts, celery, parsley and onion. Pour Mushroom Marinade over salad. Refrigerate and marinate 30 minutes before serving.

Mushroom Marinade

3 tablespoons red wine vinegar
*1½ tablespoons chopped fresh
 tarragon, or 1 teaspoon dried
 tarragon*

*freshly ground black pepper,
 to taste*
*¼ cup pure-pressed extra virgin
 olive oil*

In a small bowl, using a fork, whisk vinegar, tarragon and black pepper. Slowly drizzle in olive oil, whisking constantly until smooth. Taste, and adjust seasonings.

Pear and Gorgonzola Winter Salad

Makes 4 side-dish servings • Each serving: 9 grams protein • 10 grams carbohydrate

½ cup chopped raw walnuts

1 large head butter lettuce,
washed, dried and torn into
bite-size pieces

2 cored and sliced ripe pears

½ cup crumbled Gorgonzola
cheese

2 tablespoons chopped fresh
parsley

Winter Vinaigrette

Put walnuts in an ungreased skillet over medium-high heat. Stir nuts or shake pan almost constantly until walnuts are evenly browned and toasted. Remove from pan immediately and set aside.

Line 4 individual plates with washed and dried lettuce. Arrange pears on top. Sprinkle with Gorgonzola cheese, toasted walnuts and parsley. Spoon on Winter Vinaigrette.

Winter Vinaigrette

2 tablespoons raspberry vinegar

4 tablespoons pure-pressed extra
virgin olive oil

freshly ground black pepper,
to taste

In a small bowl, using a fork, whisk vinegar, olive oil and black pepper until smooth.

Picnic Potato Salad

Makes 6 side-dish servings • Each serving: 7 grams protein • 8 grams carbohydrate

5 medium red potatoes
  (peeled, if desired)

2 diced celery stalks

1 small diced red onion

2 tablespoons chopped fresh
  parsley

3 peeled and diced hard-boiled
  eggs* (optional)

1 diced red bell pepper

8 green beans, ends trimmed,
  sliced diagonally into 1-inch
  pieces and steamed until
  tender

Picnic Potato Salad Dressing

Boil potatoes until just barely tender, about 10 to 15 minutes. Drain and let cool. Toss potatoes and all other ingredients with Picnic Potato Salad Dressing until well coated.

Picnic Potato Salad Dressing

2 tablespoons fresh lemon juice

1 tablespoon Dijon mustard

1 egg yolk (optional)**

1 minced garlic clove

freshly ground black pepper,
  to taste

¼ cup pure-pressed extra virgin
  olive oil

2 tablespoons minced fresh chives

In a small bowl, using a fork, whisk lemon juice, mustard, egg yolk, garlic and black pepper. Slowly drizzle in oil, whisking continuously. Add chives and stir until well blended. Taste, and adjust seasonings.

*To hard boil eggs, place eggs in a medium saucepan and cover with cold water. Bring to a boil uncovered. Allow to boil for 1 minute, then cover, remove from heat and let sit undisturbed for 10 minutes. Rinse eggs under cold water. Crack shells, peel and rinse eggs.
**If you are concerned about using raw egg, omit the egg from this recipe.

Red Cabbage with Walnuts Salad

Makes 4 side-dish servings • Each serving: 5 grams protein • 3 grams carbohydrate

*1 small coarsely shredded red
  cabbage*
½ cup diced raw walnuts

2 tablespoons chopped fresh mint
Red Cabbage Vinaigrette

Combine red cabbage, walnuts and fresh mint. Toss with Red Cabbage Vinaigrette and marinate 30 minutes, refrigerated, before serving.

Red Cabbage Vinaigrette

3 tablespoons red wine vinegar
2 teaspoons Dijon mustard
*freshly ground black pepper,
  to taste*

*½ cup pure-pressed extra virgin
  olive oil*

In a small bowl, using a fork, whisk vinegar, mustard and black pepper. Slowly drizzle in olive oil, whisking constantly until smooth.

Roasted Potato, Asparagus, Red Pepper and Feta Cheese Salad

Makes 6 side-dish servings • Each serving: 8 grams protein • 25 grams carbohydrate

2 pounds red potatoes (peeled, if desired)

2 tablespoons pure-pressed extra virgin olive oil

2 minced garlic cloves

freshly ground black pepper, to taste

3 red bell peppers, roasted, or ¾ cup store-bought roasted red bell peppers

1 pound asparagus (tough ends trimmed), sliced diagonally into 1-inch pieces

1 cup diced celery stalks

½ cup slivered fresh basil, or 2 teaspoons dried basil, or ¼ cup minced fresh parsley

½ cup crumbled feta cheese

Roasted Salad Dressing (see recipe, page 171)

4 cups mixed salad greens

Preheat oven to 400°. Cut potatoes into 1-inch cubes. Toss with olive oil, garlic and black pepper. Spread potatoes evenly over a lightly greased baking sheet. Roast until browned and tender, about 20 to 30 minutes, turning occasionally. Set aside.

If using fresh red bell peppers, roast peppers directly over a gas flame or under a preheated broiler on a broiler rack. Using tongs, turn peppers frequently until blistered and blackened on all sides. Place peppers in a bowl with a plate on top. Let steam for 15 minutes to loosen skins. Peel off all charred skin. Discard skin along with seeds. Cut roasted flesh into slivers. Set aside.

Cook asparagus until just barely tender by immersing into boiling water about 3 to 6 minutes. Drain, rinse under cold water and drain again.

Gently toss roasted potatoes with bell peppers, asparagus and celery. Add fresh basil or parsley and crumbled feta cheese. Toss with Roasted Salad Dressing. Serve on a bed of salad greens.

Roasted Salad Dressing

2 tablespoons balsamic vinegar

2 teaspoons Dijon mustard

1 minced garlic clove

freshly ground black pepper,
  to taste

4 tablespoons pure-pressed extra
  virgin olive oil

In a small bowl, using a fork, whisk vinegar, mustard, garlic and black pepper. Slowly drizzle in olive oil and continue whisking until smooth and well blended.

Roasted Vegetable Salad

Makes 4 side-dish servings • Each serving: 3 grams protein 15 grams carbohydrate

1 large sweet potato, peeled and chopped into 1-inch cubes

1 cup green beans, ends trimmed, sliced diagonally into 1-inch pieces

1 tablespoon pure-pressed extra virgin olive oil

freshly ground black pepper, to taste

1 coarsely chopped red onion

1 red bell pepper, chopped into large chunks

1 tablespoon pure-pressed extra virgin olive oil

8 ounces brown or white mushrooms, stemmed and left whole

2 medium zucchini, chopped into ¼-inch rounds

1 tablespoon pure-pressed extra virgin olive oil

¼ cup balsamic vinegar

2 teaspoons Dijon mustard

¼ cup slivered fresh basil or minced parsley, for garnish

Preheat oven to 400°. Combine sweet potatoes and green beans with 1 tablespoon olive oil and black pepper. Arrange on a lightly greased baking sheet and roast, turning occasionally.

In a medium bowl, toss red onion and bell pepper with 1 table-spoon olive oil and black pepper. When sweet potatoes and beans have roasted for about 10 minutes, remove baking sheet from oven and add onion and pepper mixture, stirring well to mix. Return to oven.

While potato, bean, onion and pepper combination is roasting, combine mushrooms and zucchini and mix with 1 tablespoon olive oil and black pepper. When potato, bean, onion and pepper combination has roasted together for 5 to 10 minutes, add mushroom and zucchini mixture, stirring well to mix. Roast all together for about 5 to 10 minutes until vegetables are nicely browned and tender. Remove from oven.

In a medium serving bowl, toss all roasted vegetables with balsamic vinegar mixed with mustard. Sprinkle with chopped fresh basil or parsley. Serve at room temperature.

Russian Vegetable Salad

Makes 6 side-dish servings • Each serving: 4 grams protein • 8 grams carbohydrate

4 golden or red beets

2 large red potatoes (peeled, if desired)

½ pound green beans, ends trimmed, and sliced diagonally into 1-inch pieces

2 diced carrots

2 tablespoons minced fresh parsley

3 tablespoons drained and rinsed capers

Russian Vinaigrette

Boil whole beets in water to cover until tender, about 35 to 40 minutes. Drain and cool. Peel and dice into small cubes. Boil whole potatoes in water to cover until tender, about 25 to 30 minutes. Drain and cool. Dice into small cubes. Cook green beans and carrots in boiling water until tender, about 10 to 15 minutes. Drain and rinse under cold water.

In a large bowl, toss beets, potatoes, green beans, carrots, parsley and capers with Russian Vinaigrette.

Russian Vinaigrette

3 tablespoons balsamic vinegar

1 tablespoon Dijon mustard

freshly ground black pepper, to taste

3 tablespoons pure-pressed extra virgin olive oil

In a small bowl, using a fork, whisk balsamic vinegar, mustard and black pepper. Slowly drizzle in olive oil, whisking constantly until smooth. Pour over diced vegetables and toss gently.

Seattle Caesar Salad

Makes 4 side-dish servings • Each serving: 5 grams protein • trace carbohydrate

1 head romaine lettuce, washed,
patted dry and torn into large
pieces

Seattle Caesar Dressing

In a large serving bowl, toss washed and dried lettuce with Seattle Caesar Dressing. Serve immediately on chilled salad plates.

Seattle Caesar Dressing

2 minced garlic cloves

2 tablespoons fresh lemon juice

1 tablespoon balsamic vinegar

¼ cup pure-pressed extra virgin
olive oil

1 teaspoon Dijon mustard

1 egg yolk (optional)*

2 rinsed and coarsely chopped
anchovy fillets (optional)

6 tablespoons grated Parmesan
cheese

freshly ground black pepper,
to taste

In a blender or food processor, combine all ingredients until smooth. Taste, and adjust seasonings.

---

*If you are concerned about using raw egg, omit the egg from this recipe.

Spinach Salad with Avocado and Mushrooms

Makes 4 side-dish servings • Each serving: 7 grams protein • 8 grams carbohydrate

1 pound fresh spinach leaves, washed, dried and torn into bite-size pieces

2 ripe avocados, peeled, diced and sprinkled with fresh lemon juice

8 ounces thinly sliced brown or white mushrooms

¼ cup diced scallions

Garlic Dijon Vinaigrette

In a large serving bowl, toss all ingredients gently with Garlic Dijon Vinaigrette and serve immediately.

Garlic Dijon Vinaigrette

3 tablespoons balsamic vinegar

2 minced garlic cloves

1 tablespoon Dijon mustard

1 tablespoon slivered fresh basil, or 1 teaspoon dried basil

¾ cup pure-pressed extra virgin olive oil

freshly ground black pepper, to taste

In a blender or food processor, combine all ingredients and blend until smooth; or place ingredients in a jar with a tight-fitting lid and shake vigorously until well blended. Taste, and adjust seasonings.

Tabouli Salad

Makes 4 side-dish servings • Each serving: 8 grams protein • 24 grams carbohydrate

¾ cup bulgur wheat

1½ cups water

4 cups finely chopped fresh
   parsley

1 bunch finely chopped scallions

1 large bunch finely chopped
   fresh mint

3 medium chopped tomatoes

½ cup fresh lemon juice

½ cup pure-pressed extra virgin
   olive oil

freshly ground black pepper,
   to taste

1 head romaine lettuce, washed
   and patted dry

Pour bulgur into a bowl and cover with water. Let sit 20 minutes. Drain well, squeezing out extra water through a fine strainer or cloth. Combine drained bulgur with parsley, scallions, mint, tomatoes, lemon juice, olive oil and black pepper. Taste, and adjust seasonings.

Arrange washed and dried romaine leaves on individual plates and mound with tabouli salad.

Salad Dressings

Asian Citrus Dressing

Makes about 1 cup • 1 tablespoon: trace protein • trace carbohydrate

Use on spinach or mixed-greens salads.

1 minced garlic clove

1 teaspoon peeled and finely minced fresh ginger

2 tablespoons minced scallions

2 tablespoons fresh lime juice

2 tablespoons fresh orange juice

1 tablespoon rice wine vinegar

2 teaspoons low-sodium tamari soy sauce

¼ cup pure-pressed peanut oil

¼ cup pure-pressed sesame oil

dash cayenne pepper

In a blender or food processor, combine all ingredients and blend until smooth; or place ingredients in a jar with a tight-fitting lid and shake vigorously until well blended. Taste, and adjust seasonings. Store covered in refrigerator. Bring to room temperature before using.

Balsamic Vinaigrette

Makes about 1 cup • 1 tablespoon: trace protein • trace carbohydrate

Use on mixed-greens, spinach, marinated or roasted vegetable salads.

¼ cup balsamic vinegar

2 tablespoons fresh lemon juice

1 tablespoon Dijon mustard

2 minced garlic cloves

½ cup pure-pressed extra virgin olive oil

freshly ground black pepper, to taste

In a blender or food processor, combine all ingredients and blend until smooth; or place ingredients in a jar with a tight-fitting lid and shake vigorously until well blended. Taste, and adjust seasonings. Store covered in refrigerator. Bring to room temperature before using.

Bleu Cheese Dressing

Makes about 2 cups • 1 tablespoon: 1 gram protein • trace carbohydrate

Use on spinach, mixed-greens or potato salads.

½ cup whole sour cream

½ cup mayonnaise (made from pure-pressed oil)

⅔ cup crumbled bleu cheese

1 minced garlic clove

2 tablespoons fresh lemon juice

2 teaspoons dried basil

freshly ground black pepper, to taste

In a blender or food processor, combine all ingredients and blend until smooth; or place ingredients in a jar with a tight-fitting lid and shake vigorously until well blended. Cover and refrigerate several hours before using.

Caesar Dressing

Makes about ¾ cup • 1 tablespoon: 2 grams protein • trace carbohydrate

Use on romaine lettuce or potato salads.

2 minced garlic cloves

2 tablespoons fresh lemon juice

1 tablespoon balsamic vinegar

¼ cup pure-pressed extra virgin olive oil

1 teaspoon Dijon mustard

1 egg yolk (optional)*

2 rinsed and coarsely chopped anchovy fillets (optional)

6 tablespoons grated Parmesan cheese

freshly ground black pepper, to taste

In a blender or food processor, combine all ingredients and blend until smooth. Store covered in refrigerator.

---

*If you are concerned about using raw egg, omit the egg yolk from this recipe.

Chèvre (Goat Cheese) Dressing

Makes about 1½ cups • 1 tablespoon: 1 gram protein • trace carbohydrate

Use on roasted vegetable, mixed-greens, spinach or potato salads.

½ cup crumbled chèvre (goat cheese)

1 cup all-dairy heavy cream

1 teaspoon Dijon mustard

2 tablespoons finely chopped shallots

2 tablespoons finely slivered fresh basil, or 1 teaspoon dried basil

freshly ground black pepper, to taste

In a medium bowl, using a fork, whisk all ingredients until smooth and well blended. Taste, and adjust seasonings. Store covered in refrigerator.

Creamy Dill Dressing

Makes about 1 cup • 1 tablespoon: trace protein • trace carbohydrate

Use on mixed-greens, spinach, marinated or roasted vegetable or potato salads.

½ cup mayonnaise (made from pure-pressed oil)

½ cup whole sour cream

1 teaspoon red wine vinegar

1 tablespoon fresh lime juice

1 tablespoon minced fresh parsley

1 tablespoon minced scallions

1 tablespoon minced fresh dill, or 1 teaspoon dried dill

freshly ground black pepper, to taste

In a medium bowl, using a fork, whisk all ingredients until smooth. Taste, and adjust seasonings. Chill before using.

Creamy Vinaigrette

Makes about 1¾ cups • 1 tablespoon: trace protein • trace carbohydrate

Use on mixed-greens, marinated vegetable, spinach or potato salads.

½ cup red wine vinegar

2 tablespoons Dijon mustard

2 tablespoons fresh lemon juice

1 minced garlic clove

1 to 2 teaspoons peeled and finely minced fresh ginger (optional)

1 cup pure-pressed extra virgin olive oil

freshly ground black pepper, to taste

In a blender or food processor, combine all ingredients and blend until smooth; or place ingredients in a jar with a tight-fitting lid, and shake vigorously until well blended. Taste, and adjust seasonings. Store covered in refrigerator. Bring to room temperature before using.

French Dressing

Makes about 1½ cups • 1 tablespoon: trace protein • trace carbohydrate

Use on mixed-greens salads or marinated vegetable salads.

½ cup red wine vinegar

2 minced garlic cloves

½ teaspoon dried oregano

½ teaspoon dried basil

1 teaspoon dried tarragon

1 tablespoon Dijon mustard

freshly ground black pepper, to taste

1 cup pure-pressed extra virgin olive oil

In a small bowl, using a fork, whisk all ingredients, except olive oil. Slowly drizzle in olive oil, whisking constantly until dressing is well blended. Taste, and adjust seasonings. Store covered in refrigerator. Bring to room temperature before serving.

French Vinaigrette with Feta Cheese

Makes about 1 cup • 1 tablespoon: 1 gram protein • trace carbohydrate

Use on mixed-greens or spinach salads.

⅓ cup red wine vinegar

1 tablespoon Dijon mustard

⅓ cup pure-pressed extra virgin
   olive oil

1 tablespoon minced fresh parsley

freshly ground black pepper,
   to taste

⅓ cup crumbled feta cheese

In a small bowl, using a fork, whisk red wine vinegar and mustard. Slowly drizzle in olive oil, whisking constantly until vinaigrette thickens. Stir in parsley, black pepper and feta cheese. Taste, and adjust seasonings. Store covered in refrigerator. Bring to room temperature before using.

Garlic Vinaigrette

Makes about 1³/₄ cups • 1 tablespoon: trace protein • trace carbohydrate

Use on mixed-greens, spinach, roasted or marinated vegetable salads, or coleslaws.

5 minced garlic cloves

2 tablespoons Dijon mustard

½ cup red wine vinegar

1 cup pure-pressed extra virgin
   olive oil

¼ cup finely chopped fresh parsley

freshly ground black pepper,
   to taste

In a small bowl, using a fork, whisk garlic, mustard and vinegar until well blended. Slowly drizzle in olive oil in a steady stream, whisking until well blended. Stir in parsley. Season to taste with black pepper. Taste, and adjust seasonings. Store covered in refrigerator. Bring to room temperature before using.

Green Goddess Dressing

Makes about 1 ⅓ cups • 1 tablespoon: 1 gram protein • trace carbohydrate

Use on mixed-greens, mixed-vegetable or potato salads.

½ cup mayonnaise (made from
   pure-pressed oil)

½ cup whole sour cream

3 tablespoons all-dairy heavy
   cream

2 minced anchovy fillets
   (optional)

1 tablespoon tarragon wine
   vinegar

2 teaspoons fresh lemon juice

1 minced garlic clove

¼ cup finely chopped fresh parsley

2 tablespoons thinly sliced scallions

2 tablespoons minced fresh chives

2 tablespoons finely chopped
   fresh tarragon leaves, or
   2 teaspoons dried tarragon

freshly ground black pepper,
   to taste

In a blender or food processor, combine all ingredients and blend
until smooth; or place ingredients in a jar with a tight-fitting lid and
shake vigorously until well blended. Taste, and adjust seasonings. Store
covered in refrigerator.

Healing Oil Dressing

Makes about 1½ cups • 1 tablespoon: trace protein • trace carbohydrate

Use on mixed-greens or mixed-vegetable salads.

⅓ cup pure-pressed safflower oil

⅓ cup pure-pressed extra virgin olive oil

⅓ cup pure-pressed flaxseed oil

2 minced garlic cloves

1½ tablespoons Dijon mustard

⅓ cup balsamic vinegar

In a blender or food processor, combine all ingredients and blend until smooth; or place ingredients in a jar with a tight-fitting lid and shake vigorously until well blended. Taste, and adjust seasonings. Store covered in refrigerator. Bring to room temperature before using.

Middle Eastern Dressing

Makes about ¾ cup • 1 tablespoon: trace protein • trace carbohydrate

Use on mixed-vegetable, carrot or spinach salads, or coleslaws.

½ cup pure-pressed extra virgin olive oil

¼ cup fresh lemon or lime juice

1 minced garlic clove

2 tablespoons chopped fresh parsley

1 teaspoon grated lemon or lime zest

1 tablespoon minced scallions

1 teaspoon ground cumin

¼ teaspoon dried mustard

In a blender or food processor, combine all ingredients and blend until smooth; or place ingredients in a jar with a tight-fitting lid, and shake vigorously until well blended. Taste, and adjust seasonings. Store covered in refrigerator. Bring to room temperature before using.

Oriental Vinaigrette

Makes about 1 cup • 1 tablespoon: trace protein • trace carbohydrate

Use on vegetable salads.

¼ cup fresh lime juice

2 teaspoon grated lime zest

2 minced garlic cloves

4 teaspoons peeled and finely minced fresh ginger

¼ cup rice wine vinegar

4 teaspoons low-sodium tamari soy sauce

2 teaspoons Dijon mustard

cayenne pepper, to taste

¼ cup pure-pressed peanut oil

¼ cup pure-pressed sesame oil

In a small bowl, using a fork, whisk lime juice, lime zest, garlic, ginger, vinegar, soy sauce, mustard and cayenne pepper. Slowly whisk in peanut and sesame oils until well blended. Taste, and adjust seasonings. Store covered in refrigerator. Bring to room temperature before using.

Parmesan Salad Dressing

Makes about 1½ cups • 1 tablespoon: 1 gram protein • trace carbohydrate

Use on mixed-greens, spinach, mushroom or chef's salads.

½ cup fresh lemon juice

¾ cup pure-pressed extra virgin
 olive oil

1 tablespoon Dijon mustard

¼ cup grated Parmesan cheese

1 teaspoon dried basil

1 tablespoon chopped scallions

freshly ground black pepper,
 to taste

In a blender or food processor, combine all ingredients and blend until smooth; or place ingredients in a jar with a tight-fitting lid and shake vigorously until well blended. Taste, and adjust seasonings. Store covered in refrigerator. Bring to room temperature before using.

Ranch-Style Dressing

Makes about 1 cup • 1 tablespoon: trace protein • trace carbohydrate

Use on mixed-greens or spinach salads, or on baked potatoes.

½ cup mayonnaise (made from
 pure-pressed oil)

½ cup whole sour cream

1 minced garlic clove

1 teaspoon Dijon mustard

½ teaspoon dried dill

freshly ground black pepper,
 to taste

In a blender or food processor, combine all ingredients and blend until smooth; or place ingredients in a jar with a tight-fitting lid, and shake vigorously until well blended. Cover and refrigerate several hours before using. Taste, and adjust seasonings. Store covered in refrigerator.

Sun-Dried Tomato Vinaigrette

Makes about 1¼ cups • 1 tablespoon: trace protein • 1 gram carbohydrate

Use on mixed-greens, spinach or roasted vegetable salads.

¼ cup sun-dried tomatoes
  packed in olive oil

½ cup pure-pressed extra virgin
  olive oil

⅓ cup balsamic vinegar

2 tablespoons fresh lemon juice

2 minced garlic cloves

¼ cup slivered fresh basil, or
  2 teaspoons dried basil

2 teaspoons Dijon mustard

freshly ground black pepper,
  to taste

In a blender or food processor, combine all ingredients and blend until smooth; or place ingredients in a jar with a tight-fitting lid and shake vigorously until well blended. Add 2 to 4 tablespoons water to thin, if desired. Store covered in refrigerator. Bring to room temperature before using.

Tahini Dressing

Makes about 1 cup • 1 tablespoon: 2 grams protein • 1 gram carbohydrate

Use on mixed-greens or spinach salads.

¼ pound well-drained firm tofu, cubed (for directions, see "All You Need to Know About Tofu," page 291)

¼ cup pure-pressed vegetable oil

1 minced garlic clove

2 tablespoons fresh lemon juice

2 tablespoons sesame tahini

1 tablespoon low-sodium tamari soy sauce

1 tablespoon chopped scallions

freshly ground black pepper, to taste

2 tablespoons vegetable stock (see recipe, page 115), or canned, or water, to thin (optional)

In a blender or food processor, combine all ingredients except vegetable stock or water and blend until smooth. Thin with stock or water if desired. Taste, and adjust seasonings. Store covered in refrigerator.

Thai Vinaigrette

Makes about ¾ cup • 1 tablespoon: trace protein • trace carbohydrate

Use on mixed-greens, spinach or marinated-vegetable salads.

2 tablespoons fresh lime juice

2 tablespoons rice wine vinegar

1 tablespoon low-sodium tamari soy sauce

1 minced garlic clove

2 tablespoons minced fresh mint

2 tablespoons slivered fresh basil

2 tablespoons minced fresh cilantro

2 teaspoons peeled and finely minced fresh ginger

1 tablespoon hot chili oil

¼ cup pure-pressed extra virgin olive oil

¼ teaspoon red-pepper flakes (optional)

In a blender or food processor, combine all ingredients and blend until smooth; or place ingredients in a jar with a tight-fitting lid and shake vigorously until well blended. Cover and refrigerate several hours before using. Store covered in refrigerator.

Thousand Island Dressing

Makes about 1 ²/₃ cups • 1 tablespoon: trace protein • 1 gram carbohydrate

Use on mixed-greens or spinach salads.

*1 cup mayonnaise (made from
pure-pressed oil)*

*¼ cup chili sauce, or tomato
sauce*

¼ cup whole plain yogurt

2 tablespoons minced dill pickles

1 chopped hard-boiled egg*

*1 tablespoon finely chopped
scallions*

*1 tablespoon finely chopped fresh
parsley*

*freshly ground black pepper,
to taste*

In a medium bowl, using a fork, combine all ingredients until well mixed. Taste, and adjust seasonings. Store covered in refrigerator.

---

*To hard boil eggs, place eggs in a medium saucepan and cover with cold water. Bring to a boil uncovered. Allow to boil for 1 minute, then cover, remove from heat and let sit undisturbed 10 minutes. Rinse eggs under cold water. Crack shells, peel and rinse eggs.

Fish

Asian Shrimp and Scallops

Makes 4 servings • Each serving: 11 grams protein • 3 grams carbohydrate

12 scallops

12 raw jumbo shrimp, peeled
and deveined

1 minced garlic clove

1 teaspoon peeled and finely
minced fresh ginger

1 minced shallot

1 tablespoon sake, or mirin, or
dry sherry

2 tablespoons low-sodium tamari
soy sauce

1 tablespoon fresh lime juice

2 tablespoons pure-pressed
peanut oil

1 red bell pepper, sliced into thin
slivers

2 cups snow peas, strings
removed, ends trimmed

1 small jicama, peeled and sliced
into thin slivers; or 2 cups
sliced water chestnuts, rinsed
and drained

Topping

2 tablespoons chopped scallions

1 tablespoon chopped fresh
cilantro

½ cup dry-roasted peanuts

In a medium bowl, combine scallops, shrimp, garlic, ginger, shallots, sake, mirin, or sherry, soy sauce and lime juice. Mix well and
marinate in refrigerator at least 30 minutes. Drain well in a colander
or sieve.

In a large heavy-bottomed skillet, heat oil over medium-high heat.
When oil is hot, add marinated shrimp and scallops, bell pepper
strips, snow peas and jicama or water chestnuts. Sauté until vegetables
are brightly colored, shrimp is pink and fish is tender, about 3 to 5
minutes. Transfer to a serving platter. Sprinkle with chopped scallions,
cilantro and peanuts. Taste, and adjust seasonings.

Barbecued Whole Fish

Makes 6 servings • Each serving (not including tartar sauce):
56 grams protein • trace carbohydrate

∾

1 whole fish, about 5 pounds
  (salmon, sea bass, red snapper,
  or other firm-fleshed fish)

freshly ground black pepper,
  to taste

3 scallions cut into 2-inch
  lengths, then finely split
  lengthwise

½ cup minced celery stalks

1 tablespoon minced fresh dill, or
  1 teaspoon dried dill

1 teaspoon dried thyme

1 teaspoon dried marjoram

¼ cup minced fresh parsley

6 slices lemon

½ cup dry white wine

3 tablespoons unsalted butter

Tartar Sauce (see recipe, page
  389)

Prepare barbecue.

Rinse fish under cold water and pat dry with paper towels. Make three shallow diagonal slashes into each side of fish. Arrange on heavy-duty foil. Combine black pepper, scallions, celery, dill, thyme, marjoram and parsley. Sprinkle mixture inside fish cavity, outside on skin and inside diagonal slashes. Insert lemon slices inside fish cavity.

Pour ¼ cup of wine into cavity and dot inside of cavity with 1½ tablespoons butter. Pour remaining ¼ cup wine over fish and dot outside of fish with remaining 1½ tablespoons butter. Close foil loosely and cook over hot coals 15 to 20 minutes. Allow 10 minutes per inch thickness of fish, measured at its thickest point. Open foil and cook another 5 to 10 minutes. Serve with Tartar Sauce.

Broiled Fish with Ginger-Soy Marinade

Makes 4 servings • Each serving: 42 grams protein • trace carbohydrate

four 6-ounce fish steaks (salmon, swordfish, red snapper, sea bass, tuna or any other thick-fleshed fish)

1 minced garlic clove

1 tablespoon peeled and finely minced fresh ginger

1 tablespoon fresh lime juice

1 teaspoon grated fresh lime zest

2 to 3 tablespoons low-sodium tamari soy sauce, to taste

2 tablespoons dry sherry, or sake

2 tablespoons pure-pressed sesame oil

1 tablespoon minced fresh cilantro, or parsley

1 lime, sliced into wedges, for garnish

whole fresh cilantro or parsley sprigs, for garnish

Preheat broiler.

Rinse fish under cold water and pat dry with paper towels.

Prepare marinade by mixing garlic, ginger, lime juice, grated lime zest, soy sauce, sherry or sake, sesame oil and cilantro or parsley. Marinate fish in ginger-soy mixture about 30 minutes, turning several times. Drain fish, reserving marinade.

Broil fish steaks about 3 inches from heating element, on a lightly greased broiler pan, about 6 minutes. Turn fish, baste other side with marinade and broil another 5 minutes, until fish flakes easily with a fork. Serve garnished with lime wedges and whole cilantro or parsley sprigs.

Broiled Fish with Two Pepper Sauces

Makes 4 servings • Each serving: 42 grams protein • trace carbohydrate

2 red bell peppers or ½ cup
  store-bought roasted red bell
  peppers

2 yellow bell peppers or ½ cup
  store-bought roasted yellow
  bell peppers

¼ cup pure-pressed extra virgin
  olive oil

freshly ground black pepper,
  to taste

four 6-ounce fish steaks
  (swordfish, halibut, tuna, sea
  bass, salmon, red snapper)

pure-pressed extra virgin olive oil

freshly ground black pepper,
  to taste

fresh parsley sprigs, for garnish

If using fresh bell peppers, roast peppers directly over a gas flame or on a rack under a preheated broiler. Using tongs, turn peppers frequently, until blistered and blackened on all sides. Place peppers in a bowl with a plate on top. Let steam for 15 minutes to loosen skins. Peel off all charred skin. Discard skin along with seeds. Separate the red from the yellow peppers and coarsely chop roasted flesh. Set aside.

In a food processor, purée roasted red peppers, 2 tablespoons olive oil and black pepper. Set aside. Rinse and dry food processor. Purée the roasted yellow peppers with 2 tablespoons olive oil and black pepper. Set aside.

Preheat broiler.

Rinse fish steaks under cold water and pat dry with paper towels. Rub fish steaks with olive oil. Season to taste with black pepper. Arrange on a lightly greased broiling pan. Broil about 6 inches from heat source for 4 to 5 minutes on each side, or until fish is tender and flakes easily with a fork.

Spoon ¼ of the roasted red-pepper sauce on a heated plate. Spoon ¼ of the roasted yellow-pepper sauce next to the red sauce so that they meet in the middle. Arrange a fish steak in middle of plate over the two sauces. Repeat for remaining servings. Garnish with fresh parsley sprigs.

Cajun Blackened Fish

Makes 4 servings • Each serving: 42 grams protein • trace carbohydrate

four 6-ounce fish fillets (catfish, salmon, halibut, tuna)

1 tablespoon plus 1 teaspoon Cajun Spice Mix (homemade or store-bought)

4 tablespoons unsalted butter

1 tablespoon pure-pressed extra virgin olive oil

1 lemon, cut into wedges, for garnish

Homemade Cajun Spice Mix

1 teaspoon garlic powder

1 teaspoon dried oregano

½ teaspoon chili powder

¼ teaspoon each white pepper, black pepper and cayenne pepper

½ teaspoon dried thyme

Rinse fish under cold water and pat dry with paper towels.

If making Homemade Cajun Spice Mix, combine all ingredients in a jar and shake well to mix. Rub spice mixture on both sides of fish fillets.

In a heavy, preferably cast-iron skillet, heat butter and oil over high heat. When pan is extremely hot, add fish fillets and cook 2 to 3 minutes per side, until spices are dark and fish is opaque and flakes easily with a fork. Serve garnished with lemon wedges.

Crab or Fish Enchiladas
with Salsa Verde

Makes 8 servings • Each serving: 31 grams protein • 23 grams carbohydrate
2 tablespoons serving Mango Salsa: trace protein • 6 grams carbohydrate

Salsa Verde

2 pasilla chili peppers

8 tomatillos

2 cups water

2 minced garlic cloves

½ chopped red onion

½ cup water from cooking
tomatillos

½ cup chopped fresh cilantro

1 teaspoon dried oregano

¼ teaspoon ground cumin

cayenne pepper, to taste

½ teaspoon chili powder

1 cup whole sour cream

Prepare Salsa Verde: Roast peppers directly over a gas flame or under a preheated broiler on a broiler rack. Using tongs, turn pasilla chili peppers frequently, until blistered and blackened on all sides. Place peppers in a bowl with a plate on top. Let steam for 15 minutes to loosen skins. Peel off all charred skin. Coarsely chop roasted flesh.

Peel husks off tomatillos and rinse. In a medium saucepan, bring 2 cups water, tomatillos, garlic and onion to a boil and simmer until softened, about 15 to 20 minutes. Drain cooking water from pot, reserving ½ cup water. Transfer tomatillos, garlic, onion and reserved ½ cup water to a blender along with roasted peppers, cilantro, oregano, cumin, cayenne pepper, chili powder and sour cream. Blend until smooth. Taste, and adjust seasonings. Return to saucepan and heat to simmering. *Do not boil.* Remove from heat and set sauce aside.

Enchiladas

1¼ pounds fresh lump crabmeat;
  or 24 ounces canned crabmeat,
  drained, picked over and
  chopped; or
1¼ pounds cooked, chopped
  fish (swordfish, tuna, salmon,
  red snapper)
16 ounces crumbled Mexican-
  style cheese (queso fresco), or
  16 ounces whole cottage cheese

¼ cup minced fresh cilantro
freshly ground black pepper,
  to taste
12 corn tortillas
1½ cups grated Monterey Jack
  cheese
½ cup chopped scallions
1 cup Mango Salsa (see recipe,
  page 375)

Preheat oven to 375°.

Combine crabmeat or fish, crumbled Mexican cheese or cottage cheese, cilantro, black pepper and ½ cup salsa verde. Mix well and set aside.

Spread a thin layer of salsa verde in a greased 9 x 13-inch casserole. Using tongs, soften corn tortillas by dipping one at a time into hot sauce in saucepan for about 5 seconds. Remove from sauce and spoon 3 heaping tablespoons of filling down middle of each tortilla. Roll tortilla around filling and place seam-side down in casserole. Repeat with all tortillas. Spread remaining salsa verde sauce over filled tortillas. Sprinkle with grated cheese and chopped scallions. Bake 25 minutes, or until hot. Serve with Mango Salsa on the side.

Curry-Spiced Swordfish Kabobs

Makes 6 servings • Each serving: 39 grams protein • 2 grams carbohydrate

2 pounds swordfish, cut into
   1½-inch chunks; or any other
   thick-fleshed fish

1 cup whole plain yogurt

2 minced garlic cloves

1 teaspoon ground cumin

1 teaspoon ground coriander

2 teaspoons ground turmeric

2 tablespoons chopped fresh
   cilantro

1 teaspoon peeled and finely
   minced fresh ginger

2 tablespoons fresh lime juice

¼ to ½ teaspoon cayenne pepper,
   to taste

eight 8-inch bamboo skewers
   soaked in water 15 minutes to
   prevent burning

16 whole brown or white
   mushrooms

2 large red bell peppers, cut into
   large squares

Rinse fish under cold water and pat dry with paper towels.

In a large bowl, combine yogurt, garlic, cumin, coriander, turmeric, cilantro, ginger, lime juice and cayenne pepper. Add swordfish and coat well. Marinate at least 30 minutes or overnight, covered, in refrigerator, turning occasionally.

Prepare barbecue or preheat broiler.

Thread drained swordfish onto skewers, alternating with whole mushrooms and bell-pepper squares. Baste skewers with marinade.

Either barbecue skewers over hot coals, *or* broil skewers on a well-greased rack with a tinfoil-lined baking sheet underneath. Broil until fish is tender and cooked through, turning once, about 3 to 5 minutes per side.

Fish Tacos

Makes 8 tacos • Each taco: 31 grams protein • 18 grams carbohydrate
(Nutritional information does not include salsa)

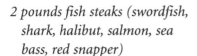

2 pounds fish steaks (swordfish, shark, halibut, salmon, sea bass, red snapper)

1 to 2 teaspoons chili powder, to taste

cayenne pepper, to taste

2 tablespoons pure-pressed extra virgin olive oil

1 tablespoon fresh lemon or lime juice

8 corn tortillas

2 cups shredded green cabbage

½ cup chopped fresh cilantro

2 sliced ripe avocados

2 chopped tomatoes

½ cup salsa (see Salsas, starting on page 374), or store-bought (no sugar added)

Rinse fish steaks under cold water and pat dry with paper towels. Cut into 1½-inch chunks. Sprinkle with chili powder and cayenne pepper.

In a large nonstick skillet, heat oil over medium high heat. When oil is hot, add fish chunks. Sauté until tender, about 5 to 7 minutes, turning occasionally. Sprinkle with lemon or lime juice.

Either layer corn tortillas between paper towels and microwave on high 10 to 20 seconds, *or* use tongs to heat tortillas directly over gas burner, turning once until softened and puffed up.

Fold a tortilla in half and fill with a portion of sautéed fish. Add cabbage, cilantro, avocado and tomato. Repeat with remaining tortillas and fillings. Top with salsa.

Greek-Style Baked Fish

Makes 4 servings • Each serving: 48 grams protein • 2 grams carbohydrate

Four 6-ounce fish steaks (swordfish, halibut, seabass, salmon)

1 red bell pepper or ¼ cup store-bought roasted red bell pepper

¼ cup pure-pressed extra virgin olive oil

2 tablespoons minced fresh parsley

1 tablespoon chopped fresh oregano or 2 teaspoons dried oregano

grated zest of 1 lemon

¼ cup fresh lemon juice

3 minced garlic cloves

1 tablespoon Dijon mustard

freshly ground black pepper, to taste

⅔ cup crumbled feta cheese

Preheat oven to 425°.

Rinse fish steaks under cold water and pat dry with paper towels.

To roast red bell pepper, place pepper in a bowl with a plate on top. Let steam for 15 minutes to loosen skin. Peel off all charred skin. Discard skin along with seeds. Dice roasted pepper.

Combine diced pepper with remaining ingredients except for feta cheese. Taste, and adjust seasonings.

Pour marinade over fish and marinate about 30 minutes, turning several times.

Arrange fish steaks in a baking dish along with marinade. Bake about 15 minutes or until fish is tender and flakes easily with a fork. Sprinkle feta cheese over top of fish during last 5 minutes of cooking.

Grilled Fish with Fresh Thai Salsa

Makes 4 servings • Each serving: 42 grams protein • trace carbohydrate

four 6-ounce fish steaks (salmon,
  swordfish, halibut, sea bass,
  red snapper or tuna)

3 tablespoons pure-pressed
  peanut oil

2 tablespoons chopped fresh
  cilantro

red-pepper flakes

1 tablespoon low-sodium tamari
  soy sauce

Fresh Thai Salsa

Rinse fish under cold water and pat dry with paper towels. Combine oil, cilantro, red-pepper flakes and soy sauce. Pour over fish and marinate at least 15 minutes.

Prepare barbecue.

Remove fish from marinade and arrange on an oiled grill 4 to 5 inches from hot coals. Grill, brushing with marinade, turning once. Allow a cooking time of about 7 to 10 minutes per inch thickness of fish. Transfer to plates and top with Fresh Thai Salsa.

Fresh Thai Salsa

3 diced tomatoes

2 tablespoons slivered fresh basil

2 teaspoons chopped fresh mint

2 tablespoons chopped fresh
  cilantro

1 tablespoon red wine vinegar

1 tablespoon fresh lime juice

2 tablespoons pure-pressed extra
  virgin olive oil

1 teaspoon low-sodium tamari
  soy sauce

1 minced garlic clove

1 tablespoon peeled and finely
  minced fresh ginger

freshly ground black pepper,
  to taste

In a large bowl, using a fork, combine all ingredients. Mix well. Taste, and adjust seasonings.

Halibut in Cream Sauce

Makes 4 servings • Each serving: 44 grams protein • trace carbohydrate

four 6-ounce halibut steaks

3 tablespoons unsalted butter

1 minced garlic clove

½ pound sliced brown or white mushrooms

grated zest of 1 lemon

2 tablespoons drained and rinsed capers

1 cup all-dairy heavy cream

freshly ground black pepper, to taste

1 tablespoon chopped fresh parsley

1 lemon cut into wedges, for garnish

Rinse halibut under cold water and pat dry with paper towels.

In a large nonstick skillet, heat butter over medium-high heat. When butter is hot and bubbly, add fish fillets and cook 2 to 3 minutes per side, or until fish flakes easily with a fork and is lightly browned. Remove and keep warm.

Add garlic and mushrooms to pan and sauté 1 minute. Add lemon zest, capers, cream, black pepper and parsley. Bring almost to a boil, reduce heat to low and simmer until sauce is slightly thickened, about 2 minutes, stirring occasionally. Taste, and adjust seasonings. Add halibut steaks and heat through. Garnish with lemon wedges and serve immediately.

Mediterranean Shrimp

Makes 4 servings • Each serving: 50 grams protein • 5 grams carbohydrate

2 tablespoons pure-pressed extra virgin olive oil

2 chopped garlic cloves

2 pounds raw shrimp, peeled and deveined

2 red or green bell peppers, cut into 1-inch squares

1 large eggplant (peeled, if desired) cut into 2-inch cubes

1 coarsely chopped medium red onion

⅓ cup pure-pressed extra virgin olive oil

freshly ground black pepper, to taste

2 medium tomatoes, cut into 1-inch cubes

1 tablespoon chopped fresh parsley

1 tablespoon fresh lemon juice

⅓ cup crumbled feta cheese

Preheat oven to 425°.

In a large nonstick skillet, heat oil over medium-high heat. When oil is hot, add garlic and shrimp and cook 2 to 5 minutes, or until shrimp are tender and turn pink. Remove from heat and set aside.

In a large bowl, combine bell pepper, eggplant, onion, olive oil and black pepper. Transfer to a greased baking sheet, spread in a single layer, and roast, stirring occasionally, until all vegetables are tender, about 20 minutes. Add tomatoes the last 5 minutes. Arrange all vegetables on a serving platter. Top with shrimp, parsley, lemon juice and crumbled feta cheese. Taste, and adjust seasonings. Serve hot or at room temperature.

Oven-Steamed Asian-Style Fish

Makes 4 servings • Each serving: 43 grams protein • trace carbohydrate

four 6-ounce thick fish fillets (halibut, salmon, swordfish, red snapper, cod, or sea bass)

2 cups sliced brown or white mushrooms

2 tablespoons low-sodium tamari soy sauce

2 tablespoons dry sherry

1 tablespoon pure-pressed sesame oil

1 tablespoon fresh lime juice

⅓ cup chopped fresh scallions

1 tablespoon chopped fresh mint

2 tablespoons chopped fresh cilantro

2 minced garlic cloves

2 teaspoons peeled and finely minced fresh ginger

cayenne pepper, to taste

1 lime cut into wedges, for garnish

4 fresh cilantro sprigs, for garnish

Rinse fish under cold water and pat dry with paper towels. Arrange fish fillets in a greased baking dish. Top with sliced mushrooms.

In a small bowl, combine soy sauce, sherry, sesame oil, lime juice, scallions, mint, cilantro, garlic and ginger. Season to taste with cayenne pepper. Pour over fish and marinate at least 30 minutes.

Preheat oven to 375°. Bake, covered with foil, until fish turns opaque and flakes easily with a fork, about 20 minutes. Garnish with fresh lime wedges and cilantro sprigs and serve immediately.

Pan-Fried Trout Amandine

Makes 4 servings • Each serving: 44 grams protein • 6 grams carbohydrate

four 6-ounce trout fillets

1 thinly sliced lemon

8 fresh sprigs thyme

freshly ground black pepper,
to taste

1 teaspoon paprika

¼ cup flour

2 tablespoons unsalted butter

2 tablespoons pure-pressed extra
virgin olive oil

2 tablespoons sliced raw almonds

1 tablespoon fresh lemon juice

1 tablespoon chopped fresh
parsley

Rinse trout under cold water and pat dry with paper towels. Insert lemon slices and fresh thyme sprigs into cavity of fish. In a shallow dish, mix black pepper, paprika and flour. Dredge each fish lightly in flour mixture, being careful not to spill herbs and lemons from the cavity.

In a large heavy-bottomed nonstick skillet, heat butter and oil over medium-high heat. When hot, add trout and cook 3 to 5 minutes per side, or until tender and flesh flakes easily with a fork. Shake pan to prevent sticking.

Remove fish from pan and keep warm. Add almonds and lemon juice, and cook two minutes, stirring occasionally. Pour over fish and sprinkle with chopped parsley.

Parchment-Baked Fish

Makes 4 servings • Each serving: 42 grams protein • 2 grams carbohydrate

four 6-ounce fish steaks (salmon, halibut, sea bass, red snapper, swordfish, tuna or other thick-fleshed fish)

2 teaspoons grated fresh lemon zest

4 tablespoons chopped mixed fresh herbs (any combination of oregano, basil, parsley, chives, tarragon)

freshly ground black pepper, to taste

4 tablespoons dry white wine, or vermouth

4 tablespoons melted unsalted butter

1 tablespoon Dijon mustard

1 lemon cut into wedges, for garnish

Preheat oven to 375°.

Rinse fish under cold water and pat dry with paper towels. Arrange each fish steak on a sheet of parchment baking paper or a double sheet of foil. Sprinkle with lemon zest, fresh herbs and black pepper. Combine wine or vermouth, butter and mustard and pour over fish, making sure that edges of paper are folded up to hold sauce. Tightly seal packets by double-folding edges and sides. Arrange on a baking sheet and bake about 15 minutes, until fish is tender and easily flakes with a fork. Garnish with fresh lemon wedges and serve immediately.

Poached Salmon with Garlic Mayonnaise

Makes 4 servings • Each serving: 42 grams protein • trace carbohydrate

four 6-ounce salmon steaks

fish stock (see recipe, page 114),
   or ½ water, ½ white wine,
   to cover

4 lemon slices

Garlic Mayonnaise

Rinse salmon steaks under cold water and pat dry with paper towels. In a large skillet, cover salmon with fish stock or ½ water and ½ white wine to totally immerse fish. Add lemon slices and bring to a boil. Reduce heat and simmer gently until tender, or until fish flakes easily with a fork, about 10 to 15 minutes. Remove fish carefully with one or two spatulas. Drain well and serve with Garlic Mayonnaise.

Garlic Mayonnaise

1 egg yolk*

2 tablespoons fresh lemon juice

1 teaspoon grated lemon zest

1 minced garlic clove

1 teaspoon capers, drained and
   rinsed

freshly ground black pepper,
   to taste

¼ cup pure-pressed extra virgin
   olive oil

¼ cup pure-pressed canola oil

1 tablespoon minced fresh parsley

In a blender, combine egg yolk, lemon juice, lemon zest, garlic, capers and black pepper. With motor running, gradually add oils, blending until sauce is smooth and creamy. Remove to a bowl and stir in parsley. Taste, and adjust seasonings.

Makes about ¾ cup.

———————

*If you are concerned about using raw egg, choose an alternate recipe.

Red Snapper Veracruz

Makes 4 servings • Each serving: 56 grams protein • trace carbohydrate

2 pounds red snapper fillets

1 tablespoon fresh lime juice

freshly ground black pepper, to taste

2 tablespoons pure-pressed extra virgin olive oil

1 medium thinly sliced red onion

4 minced garlic cloves

1 thinly sliced green bell pepper

1 small minced fresh jalapeño pepper; or 1 to 2 tablespoons canned diced green chilies, to taste [wear rubber gloves to prepare fresh jalapeño pepper]

2 medium peeled, seeded and chopped tomatoes*

¼ cup sliced green olives

1 tablespoon drained and rinsed capers

Preheat oven to 450°.

Rinse red snapper under cold water and pat dry with paper towels. Sprinkle fish with lime juice and black pepper and set aside.

In a large nonstick skillet, heat oil over medium-high heat. When oil is hot, add onion, garlic, bell pepper and jalapeño pepper and sauté until softened, about 5 minutes. Add tomatoes, green olives and capers and cook until heated through. Taste, and adjust seasonings.

Pour ½ of sauce in a greased 9×13-inch baking pan. Arrange red snapper fillets on top of the sauce. Spread remaining sauce over fish. Cover and bake until fish is tender and flakes easily with a fork, about 8 to 10 minutes.

---

*To peel and seed tomatoes: Plunge tomatoes into boiling water for several seconds, then into cold water. The skins will slip off easily. Cut tomatoes in half and squeeze gently. Scoop out seeds using a small spoon or your fingers. Chop tomatoes.

Santa Barbara Shrimp Sauté

Makes 4 servings • Each serving: 47 grams protein • trace carbohydrate

2 tablespoons unsalted butter

2 tablespoons pure-pressed extra virgin olive oil

3 minced garlic cloves

2 cups asparagus, tough ends trimmed, and sliced diagonally into 1-inch pieces; or 2 cups green beans, ends trimmed, and sliced diagonally into 1-inch pieces

2 cups sliced brown or white mushrooms

2 pounds raw shrimp, peeled and deveined

2 tablespoons fresh lime juice

1 tablespoon chopped fresh parsley

freshly ground black pepper, to taste

In a large nonstick skillet, heat butter and oil over medium-high heat. When hot, add garlic, asparagus or green beans and mushrooms and sauté until almost tender, about 5 to 7 minutes. Add shrimp and sauté until tender and pink, about 3 to 5 minutes. Stir in lime juice, parsley and black pepper. Taste, and adjust seasonings.

Shrimp and Roasted Peppers

Makes 4 servings • Each serving: 47 grams protein • trace carbohydrate

2 pounds raw large shrimp

3 red bell peppers or ¾ cup
  store-bought roasted red bell
  peppers

1 tablespoon minced chives

1 tablespoon balsamic vinegar

1 tablespoon pure-pressed extra
  virgin olive oil

freshly ground black pepper,
  to taste

2 cups fresh spinach, washed,
  stemmed and torn into
  bite-size pieces

In a large pot, bring 2 quarts of water to a boil. Add shrimp. Reduce heat to low and simmer 2 to 3 minutes, until shrimp turn pink. Using a slotted spoon, remove from boiling water. Rinse immediately under cold water for 2 minutes. Peel shrimp and devein by slicing along back ridge with a small sharp knife and carefully lifting out the black vein.

If using fresh red bell peppers, roast peppers directly over a gas flame or on a rack under a preheated broiler. Using tongs, turn peppers frequently until blistered and blackened on all sides. Place peppers in a bowl with a plate on top. Let steam for 15 minutes to loosen skin. Peel off all charred skin. Discard skin along with seeds. Cut roasted flesh into thin slivers.

In a large bowl, combine shrimp, roasted bell peppers, chives, vinegar, olive oil and black pepper, to taste. Arrange spinach on a serving platter. Mound with shrimp mixture. Serve chilled.

Sole Amandine
with Caper-Butter Sauce

Makes 4 servings • Each serving: 45 grams protein • 8 grams carbohydrate

⅓ cup slivered raw almonds,
  for garnish

four 6-ounce sole fillets

¼ cup flour

freshly ground black pepper,
  to taste

6 tablespoons unsalted butter

1 tablespoon drained and rinsed
  capers

juice of 1 lemon

1 tablespoon chopped fresh
  parsley, for garnish

Put almonds in an ungreased skillet over medium-high heat. Stir nuts or shake pan almost constantly, until almonds are evenly browned and toasted. Remove from pan immediately and set aside.

Rinse sole fillets under cold water and pat dry with paper towels. Mix flour and black pepper in a brown paper bag. Add fish fillets, one at a time, and shake well, until lightly dredged. Repeat until all fish are well coated with flour mixture.

In a large nonstick skillet, heat 3 tablespoons butter over medium-high heat. When butter is hot and bubbly, add fish and sauté until lightly browned, turning once, about 2 to 3 minutes per side. Transfer fish from pan onto a heat-proof platter and keep warm in a low oven.

Heat remaining 3 tablespoons butter over medium heat until melted and foaming. Add capers and lemon juice and cook until heated through, about 1 minute. *Do not brown.* Pour over fish. Sprinkle with chopped parsley and toasted slivered almonds.

Spanish Halibut

Makes 4 servings • Each serving: 42 grams protein • trace carbohydrate

four 6-ounce halibut fillets

6 tablespoons red wine vinegar

¼ teaspoon crushed saffron

1 thinly sliced red bell pepper

2 minced shallots

2 minced garlic cloves

1 tablespoon pure-pressed extra virgin olive oil

1 teaspoon dried thyme

1 tablespoon minced fresh parsley

freshly ground black pepper, to taste

Rinse halibut under cold water and pat dry with paper towels.

In a large nonstick skillet bring about 1 inch of water to a simmer over medium heat. Stir in 4 tablespoons of vinegar and the saffron. Add halibut fillets and bell pepper. Simmer until fish flakes easily with a fork, about 15 minutes. Using a slotted spatula, carefully remove fish and bell peppers. Drain and transfer to a serving dish.

In a medium bowl, combine remaining 2 tablespoons vinegar with shallots, garlic, olive oil, thyme, parsley and black pepper. Taste, and adjust seasonings. Pour over fish, cover and refrigerate at least 1 hour. Serve cold or at room temperature.

Steamed Clams

Makes 4 servings • Each serving: 18 grams protein • trace carbohydrate

5 dozen clams

½ cup dry white wine

½ cup water

4 chopped garlic cloves

2 chopped shallots

2 bay leaves

2 sprigs fresh thyme, or
 1 teaspoon dried thyme

6 peppercorns

Scrub clams until all grit is removed. In a deep pot, bring clams and remaining ingredients to a boil and cook over high heat. Keep pot tightly covered until all clams have opened, about 3 to 10 minutes, depending on size. Occasionally shake pot to redistribute clams. Remove opened clams from pot. Discard any clams that did not open. Strain broth and serve on the side in a small bowl. Dip clams in either broth or garlic butter.

Garlic Butter

1 stick (½ cup) unsalted butter

3 to 4 minced garlic cloves

1 tablespoon minced fresh parsley

In a small saucepan, melt butter. Stir in garlic and parsley. Serve immediately.

Swordfish and Pineapple Brochettes

Makes 4 servings • Each serving: 57 grams protein • 17 grams carbohydrate

2 red or green bell peppers

1 small pineapple

⅓ cup fresh orange juice

¼ cup peeled chopped fresh ginger

1 tablespoon low-sodium tamari soy sauce

four 8-ounce swordfish steaks

eight 8-inch skewers soaked in water 15 minutes to prevent burning

3 tablespoons mayonnaise (made from pure-pressed oil)

1 teaspoon curry powder

dash cayenne pepper, to taste

Cut bell peppers in sixteen 1-inch squares. Set aside.

Peel and core pineapple. Slice into 1-inch-thick round-slices and then cut into twenty-four 1-inch cubes. Set aside. Coarsely chop remaining pineapple and place in a blender with orange juice, fresh ginger and soy sauce. Purée until smooth. Pour into a medium bowl.

Rinse swordfish under cold water and pat dry with paper towels. Cut swordfish into 1-inch cubes. Pour ½ of pineapple purée over fish and coat well. Cover and marinate in refrigerator 1 hour.

Preheat broiler.

Alternate 3 swordfish cubes and 2 bell pepper squares with 3 pineapple cubes on each skewer. Arrange skewers on a lightly greased broiler pan, or a greased rack with a tinfoil-lined baking sheet underneath. Broil about 4 inches from heat source, turning to broil evenly on all sides, about 10 minutes.

In a small saucepan, heat reserved marinade, bringing it to a boil. Remove from heat and whisk in mayonnaise, curry powder and cayenne pepper until smooth. Pour on top of brochettes before serving.

Thai Shrimp Curry

Makes 4 servings • Each serving: 30 grams protein • 2 grams carbohydrate

2 tablespoons pure-pressed
   peanut oil

1 medium minced onion

3 minced garlic cloves

1 teaspoon ground cumin

1 teaspoon ground coriander

1 teaspoon ground turmeric

¼ teaspoon red-pepper flakes

1¼ pounds raw shrimp, peeled
   and deveined

1½ tablespoons low-sodium
   tamari soy sauce

2 tablespoons fresh lime juice

2 tablespoons dry-roasted, finely
   chopped peanuts or cashews,
   for garnish

1 tablespoon chopped fresh
   cilantro, for garnish

In a wok or a large nonstick skillet, heat oil over medium-high heat. When oil is hot, add onion, garlic, cumin, coriander, turmeric and red pepper flakes, and stir-fry until softened, about 5 minutes. Add shrimp and soy sauce and stir-fry until shrimp are tender and pink, about 2 to 3 minutes. Add lime juice. Sprinkle with peanuts or cashews and cilantro. Taste, and adjust seasonings.

Chicken and Turkey

Chicken Breast Piccata

Makes 4 servings • Each serving: 67 grams protein • 37 grams carbohydrate

2 pounds skinless, boneless
chicken breasts

2 cups fresh or dried whole-grain
bread crumbs

2 teaspoons dried oregano

2 tablespoons minced fresh parsley

2 teaspoons dried basil

freshly ground black pepper,
to taste

2 eggs

2 tablespoons pure-pressed extra
virgin olive oil

½ cup white wine

½ cup chicken stock (see recipe,
page 113), or low-sodium
canned

3 tablespoons fresh lemon juice

2 tablespoons rinsed and drained
capers

1 tablespoon minced fresh parsley

Rinse chicken breasts under cold water and pat dry with paper towels. Place each breast between two sheets of waxed paper or plastic wrap. Pound to ¼ inch thickness, using a heavy mallet or the back of a skillet. Trim ragged edges.

In a shallow dish, mix bread crumbs, oregano, parsley, basil and black pepper. In a separate shallow dish, beat eggs. Dip each flattened chicken breast into beaten egg and then into seasoned bread crumbs, coating completely.

In a large nonstick skillet, heat oil over medium-high heat. When oil is hot, reduce heat to medium. Add chicken breasts, in batches, if necessary, and sauté until golden brown and tender, about 3 to 5 minutes on each side. Remove chicken breasts to a heat-proof platter and keep warm in preheated oven.

Add wine to skillet and let simmer, scraping bottom of pan to mix in bits of chicken stuck to pan. Add chicken stock, lemon juice and capers.

Bring to a boil, reduce heat to low and simmer 15 minutes. Taste, and adjust seasonings. Pour sauce over breasts and garnish with minced parsley. Serve immediately.

Chicken Cordon Bleu

Makes 6 servings • Each serving: 49 grams protein • trace carbohydrate

2 pounds skinless, boneless
  chicken breasts

6 thin slices nitrate-free ham

6 thin slices Gruyère cheese

2 tablespoons unsalted butter

2 tablespoons pure-pressed extra
  virgin olive oil

freshly ground black pepper,
  to taste

½ cup chopped shallots

2 cups sliced brown or white
  mushrooms

½ cup dry white wine

½ cup all-dairy heavy cream

1 tablespoon chopped fresh
  parsley, for garnish

Rinse chicken under cold water and pat dry with paper towels. Place each breast between two sheets of waxed paper or plastic wrap. Pound to ¼-inch thickness using a heavy mallet or back of a skillet. Trim ragged edges.

Lay a flattened chicken breast on your work surface. Top with a slice of ham and a slice of cheese. Roll, jelly-roll style, and secure with a wooden toothpick. Repeat with remaining breasts.

In a large nonstick skillet, heat butter and olive oil over medium-high heat. When hot, add chicken roll-ups and cook until lightly browned and tender, about 10 to 12 minutes. Season to taste with black pepper. Remove chicken from pan and keep warm.

To pan drippings add shallots and mushrooms. Sauté until softened, about 5 minutes. Add white wine and simmer 3 minutes. Add cream and stir well. Arrange chicken rolls in pan. Heat slowly (do not boil), turning occasionally, about 3 minutes, until heated through. Taste, and adjust seasonings. Sprinkle with chopped parsley and serve.

Chicken Creole Style

Makes 4 servings • Each serving: 56 grams protein • trace carbohydrate

2 pounds boneless chicken breasts

½ cup pure-pressed extra virgin
olive oil

1½ tablespoons dry sherry

1 teaspoon dried oregano

½ teaspoon ground cumin

2 tablespoons chopped shallots

2 minced garlic cloves

2 tablespoons minced fresh
parsley

freshly ground black pepper,
to taste

Rinse chicken under cold water and pat dry with paper towels.

In a shallow dish, combine olive oil, sherry, oregano, cumin, shallots, garlic, parsley and black pepper. Add chicken pieces and coat each piece completely. Marinate 1 to 3 hours, if possible.

Preheat oven to 350°. Arrange chicken in a greased baking dish and bake until chicken is tender and juicy, about 30 minutes, basting frequently with marinade. Taste, and adjust seasonings.

Chicken Fajitas

Makes 4 servings • Each serving: 63 grams protein • 35 grams carbohydrate
(Nutritional information does not include salsa)

2 pounds skinless, boneless
  chicken breasts or thighs

2 tablespoons fresh lime juice

2 minced garlic cloves

2 teaspoons chili powder

freshly ground black pepper,
  to taste

2 tablespoons pure-pressed extra
  virgin olive oil

1 thinly sliced medium red onion

2 thinly sliced red or green bell
  peppers

1 small diced fresh jalapeño
  pepper; or 1 to 2 tablespoons
  canned diced green peppers
  [wear rubber gloves to
  prepare fresh jalapeño pepper]

8 corn tortillas

Topping

1 cup Guacamole (see recipe,
  page 93)

½ cup whole sour cream

½ cup salsa (see Salsas, starting
  on page 374), or store-bought
  (no sugar added)

2 tablespoons chopped fresh
  cilantro

Rinse chicken under cold water and pat dry with paper towels. Cut chicken into strips. In a medium bowl, combine lime juice, garlic, chili powder, black pepper and chicken strips. Allow to marinate while preparing remaining ingredients.

In a large nonstick skillet, heat oil over medium-high heat. When oil is hot, add onion, bell pepper and jalapeño pepper. Cook until softened, about 5 minutes. Drain chicken strips and add to skillet. Sauté until chicken is tender, about 10 minutes, stirring occasionally.

Either layer corn tortillas between paper towels and microwave on high 10 to 20 seconds, or use tongs to heat tortillas directly over gas burner, turning once until softened and puffed up.

Spoon chicken mixture into warmed corn tortillas. Top with guacamole, sour cream, salsa and cilantro.

Chicken Fricassee

Makes 4 servings • Each serving: 61 grams protein • 15 grams carbohydrate
½ cup Basic Steamed Brown Rice: 3 grams protein • 24 grams carbohydrate
½ cup Garlic Mashed Potatoes: 3 grams protein • 26 grams carbohydrate

2 tablespoons pure-pressed extra virgin olive oil

2 tablespoons unsalted butter

1 large diced onion

4 minced garlic cloves

2 pounds boneless chicken breasts, diced

2 cups sliced brown or white mushrooms

one 13¾-ounce can artichoke hearts, packed in water, drained, rinsed and diced

freshly ground black pepper, to taste

dash to ¼ teaspoon cayenne pepper, to taste

1½ cups all-dairy heavy cream

2 tablespoons Dijon mustard

1 cup fresh green peas, steamed or frozen and thawed

2 tablespoons chopped fresh parsley, for garnish

In a large saucepan, heat butter and oil over medium-high heat. When hot, add onion and garlic and sauté until softened, about 5 minutes. Add diced chicken to saucepan and sauté until barely tender, about 5 minutes. Add mushrooms, artichoke hearts, black pepper and cayenne pepper and mix well.

Add cream and mustard and simmer over low heat until reduced to a creamy consistency, about 15 minutes. *Do not boil.* Add peas, taste, and adjust seasonings. Garnish with chopped parsley. Serve over Basic Steamed Brown Rice (page 320) or Garlic Mashed Potatoes (page 355).

Chicken in Sour Cream

Makes 4 servings • Each serving: 64 grams protein • 18 grams carbohydrate
½ cup Basic Steamed Brown Rice: 3 grams protein • 24 grams carbohydrate
½ cup Garlic Mashed Potatoes: 3 grams protein • 26 grams carbohydrate

*2 pounds boneless chicken breasts
 or thighs*

⅓ cup unsalted butter

1 medium chopped onion

2 minced garlic cloves

1 chopped red or green bell pepper

*2 cups sliced brown or white
 mushrooms*

*freshly ground black pepper,
 to taste*

3 tablespoons flour

*1 cup chicken stock (see recipe,
 page 113),* or *low-sodium
 canned, heated until simmering*

1 cup fresh green peas or *frozen
 and thawed*

2 cups whole sour cream

1 tablespoon fresh lemon juice

1 teaspoon grated lemon zest

*2 tablespoons chopped fresh
 parsley*

Rinse chicken under cold water and pat dry with paper towels. Cut into chunks.

In a large nonstick skillet, melt butter over medium-high heat. When butter is hot and bubbly, add onion, garlic and bell pepper and cook over medium heat until softened, about 5 minutes. Add chicken pieces, mushrooms and black pepper and cook, turning frequently, about 10 minutes. Reduce heat to low. Cover and simmer until chicken is tender, about 15 minutes. Transfer chicken and vegetables to a platter. Cover with foil and keep warm in a preheated oven.

Add flour to pan drippings. Cook over medium heat 2 minutes, stirring constantly. Whisk in the heated chicken stock, stirring until smooth. Bring to a boil. Reduce heat to low and simmer until thickened, about 2 minutes. Add peas and sour cream and stir until well blended and creamy. Add lemon juice, lemon zest and parsley. Combine chicken and vegetables with sour cream sauce. Cook until chicken is heated through. *Do not boil.* Taste, and adjust seasonings. Serve over Basic Steamed Brown Rice (page 320) or Garlic Mashed Potatoes (page 355).

Chicken Parmesan

Makes 4 servings • Each serving: 86 grams protein • 25 grams carbohydrate

2 pounds skinless, boneless
  chicken breasts

1½ cups fresh or dried whole-
  grain bread crumbs

½ cup grated Parmesan cheese

2 teaspoons dried oregano

2 teaspoons dried basil

2 tablespoons minced fresh parsley

freshly ground black pepper,
  to taste

2 beaten eggs

2 tablespoons pure-pressed extra
  virgin olive oil

3 cups Basic Tomato Sauce,
  (see recipe, page 378), or
  store-bought (no sugar added)

½ pound grated mozzarella
  cheese

2 tablespoons grated Parmesan
  cheese

Preheat oven to 350°. Rinse chicken under cold water and pat dry with paper towels. Place chicken between two pieces of waxed paper or plastic wrap. Pound to ¼-inch thickness using a heavy mallet or back of a skillet. Trim ragged edges.

In a shallow bowl, combine bread crumbs, Parmesan cheese, oregano, basil, parsley and black pepper.

In a separate shallow bowl, beat eggs. Dip chicken first in egg, then in seasoned crumb mixture until well coated.

In a large nonstick skillet, heat oil over medium-high heat. When oil is hot, add chicken breasts and sauté until lightly browned, about 5 minutes per side. Arrange chicken in a single layer in a 9×13-inch lightly greased baking dish. Pour tomato sauce over chicken. Top with mozzarella cheese. Bake 15 to 20 minutes or until hot and bubbly. Sprinkle with Parmesan cheese before serving.

Chicken Provençal

Makes 6 servings • Each serving: 56 grams protein • 7 grams carbohydrate

3 pounds chicken pieces

Marinade

*1 tablespoon pure-pressed extra
virgin olive oil*

1 tablespoon fresh lemon juice

*freshly ground black pepper,
to taste*

Provençal Sauce

*2 tablespoons pure-pressed extra
virgin olive oil*

*1 medium red onion, cut into
thin strips*

3 minced garlic cloves

*1 green or red bell pepper, sliced
into thin strips*

*28 ounces canned Italian plum
tomatoes with basil, drained
and coarsely chopped
(reserve liquid)*

2 teaspoons grated orange zest

*½ cup Pernod (anise liqueur), or
red wine*

*1 tablespoon Herbes de Provence
(or combination of lavender,
rosemary and fennel)*

2 teaspoons dried thyme

*freshly ground black pepper,
to taste*

*2 tablespoons minced fresh
parsley, for garnish*

Rinse chicken under cold water and pat dry with paper towels. Place in a shallow dish. In a small bowl, combine 1 tablespoon olive oil, lemon juice and black pepper. Pour over chicken pieces and set aside to marinate 1 hour, refrigerated.

In a large saucepan, heat 2 tablespoons olive oil over medium-high heat. When oil is hot, add onion, garlic and bell pepper and sauté until softened, about 5 minutes. Add tomatoes and their liquid, orange zest, liqueur, or red wine, Herbes de Provence, thyme and black pepper. Bring to a boil. Reduce heat and simmer, partially covered, 35 to 40 minutes. Taste, and adjust seasonings.

Preheat broiler.

Arrange chicken on a greased rack with a tinfoil-lined baking sheet underneath. Broil chicken until browned on outside and tender inside, turning once and brushing with leftover marinade. Transfer chicken to individual plates. Top with Provençal Sauce. Garnish with minced parsley.

Chicken Tacos

Makes 4 servings • Each taco: 41 grams protein • 34 grams carbohydrate
(Nutritional information does not include salsa)

1 tablespoon pure-pressed extra
   virgin olive oil

1 minced garlic clove

1 medium chopped red onion

1 chopped red or green bell pepper

½ teaspoon ground cumin

½ teaspoon dried oregano

freshly ground black pepper,
   to taste

1 tablespoon pure-pressed extra
   virgin olive oil

4 boneless skinless chicken
   breasts, diced

8 corn tortillas

Topping

1 cup grated Monterey Jack cheese

¼ cup minced fresh cilantro

¼ cup minced scallions

1 cup chopped tomatoes

1 sliced ripe avocado

2 cups shredded lettuce

1 cup salsa (see Salsas, starting
   on page 374), or store-bought
   (no sugar added)

In a large nonstick skillet, heat 1 tablespoon oil over medium-high heat. When oil is hot, add garlic, onion, bell pepper, cumin, oregano and black pepper and sauté until softened, about 5 minutes. Remove from pan and set aside. Heat remaining 1 tablespoon oil in same skillet over medium-high heat. When oil is hot, add diced chicken and sauté until chicken is tender, about 5 to 10 minutes. Add sautéed vegetables to cooked chicken and cook until heated through.

Either layer corn tortillas between paper towels and microwave on high 10 or 20 seconds, *or* use tongs to heat tortillas directly over gas burner, turning once until softened and puffed up.

Spoon chicken and vegetable mixture onto tortillas, dividing evenly. Fold each taco in half and top with grated cheese, cilantro, scallions, tomatoes, avocado and lettuce. Serve salsa on the side.

Chicken Torta

Makes 4 servings • Each serving: 53 grams protein • 22 grams carbohydrate

1 pound skinless, boneless
   chicken breasts

2 tablespoons pure-pressed extra
   virgin olive oil

1 small chopped onion

2 minced garlic cloves

1 chopped red bell pepper

1 tablespoon minced fresh
   rosemary or 1 teaspoon dried
   rosemary

8 eggs

1½ cups cooked rice

¼ cup slivered fresh basil or
   2 teaspoons dried basil

6½ ounce jar marinated
   artichoke hearts or mushrooms,
   drained and chopped

⅔ cup crumbled feta cheese

1 teaspoon grated lemon zest

freshly ground black pepper,
   to taste

2 tablespoons finely minced fresh
   parsley

Preheat oven to 375°.

Rinse chicken under cold water and pat dry with paper towels. Cut into 1-inch chunks.

In a large nonstick skillet heat oil over medium-high heat. When oil is hot, add onion, garlic and bell pepper. Sauté 5 minutes, stirring often. Add chicken and rosemary and sauté 5 more minutes. Remove from heat, drain excess liquid and set chicken and vegetable mixture aside.

In a large bowl, using a fork, whisk eggs. Add rice, basil, artichoke hearts or mushrooms, feta cheese, lemon zest and black pepper. Mix well. Add chicken and vegetable mixture and stir until well blended.

Pour into a 10-inch lightly greased ovenproof dish. Bake about 45 minutes until eggs are set. Cool 15 minutes before slicing. Garnish with minced parsley.

Chicken with Mustard Sour Cream Sauce

Makes 4 servings • Each serving: 58 grams protein • 3 grams carbohydrate

2 pounds boneless chicken breasts

2 tablespoons pure-pressed extra virgin olive oil

¼ cup fresh lime juice

2 minced garlic cloves

¼ cup minced fresh cilantro

freshly ground black pepper, to taste

2 tablespoons pure-pressed extra virgin olive oil

¼ cup Dijon mustard

¼ cup drained and rinsed capers

1 cup whole sour cream

1 tablespoon finely chopped scallions

1 to 2 tablespoons fresh lime juice, to taste

dash cayenne pepper

4 whole fresh cilantro sprigs, for garnish

Rinse chicken breasts under cold water and pat dry with paper towels. In a shallow dish, combine 2 tablespoons olive oil, ¼ cup lime juice, garlic, cilantro and black pepper. Add chicken breasts and marinate at least 30 minutes.

In a large nonstick skillet, heat remaining 2 tablespoons oil over medium-high heat. When oil is hot, add chicken and sauté over medium heat until browned on both sides and cooked through about 5 minutes per side. Transfer from pan onto a heat-proof platter and keep warm in a preheated oven.

Using a slotted spoon, remove any remaining chicken bits from pan, leaving the juices. Using a fork, whisk in mustard, capers, sour cream and scallions. Cook until heated through over low heat. *Do not boil.* Add additional 1 to 2 tablespoons lime juice and cayenne pepper. Taste, and adjust seasonings. Pour sauce over chicken and serve garnished with whole cilantro sprigs.

Curried Chicken

Makes 6 servings • Each serving: 57 grams protein • 2 grams carbohydrate

3 pounds chicken pieces

2 tablespoons pure-pressed
peanut oil

2 tablespoons unsalted butter

1 large chopped onion

2 minced garlic cloves

2 chopped red or green bell
peppers

1 tablespoon peeled and finely
minced fresh ginger

1 tablespoon curry powder

½ teaspoon paprika

freshly ground black pepper,
to taste

¼ cup chicken stock (see recipe,
page 113), or low-sodium
canned or water

1 cup whole sour cream

1 tablespoon chopped fresh
cilantro, for garnish

Rinse chicken under cold water and pat dry with paper towels.

In a large nonstick skillet, heat oil over medium-high heat. When oil is hot, add chicken and sauté over medium heat until browned on both sides, about 5 minutes per side. Remove from pan, drain well and set aside. Wipe out skillet with a paper towel.

In the same skillet, melt butter over medium-high heat. When butter is hot and bubbly, add onion, garlic and bell pepper and sauté until softened, about 5 minutes. Reduce heat to medium and add ginger, curry powder, paprika and black pepper. Stir well. Add chicken pieces and stock or water. Bring to a boil. Reduce heat to low. Add sour cream and mix well. Cover and simmer over low heat until chicken is tender, about 20 to 30 minutes, stirring occasionally. Taste, and adjust seasonings. Sprinkle with chopped cilantro.

Enchiladas Suizas

Makes 6 servings • Each serving: 29 grams protein • 30 grams carbohydrate

Salsa Verde

1 pound tomatillos, husked and quartered

2 chopped garlic cloves

½ small chopped red onion

1 small chopped fresh jalapeño pepper; or *1 to 2 tablespoons canned diced green chilies, to taste* [wear rubber gloves to prepare fresh jalapeño peppers]

1¾ cups chicken stock (see recipe, page 113), or *low-sodium canned*

1 cup whole sour cream

freshly ground black pepper, to taste

Prepare Salsa Verde: In a medium saucepan, bring tomatillos, garlic, onion, jalapeño pepper and chicken stock to a boil over medium-high heat. Reduce heat to low and simmer until tomatillos and onion are soft, about 20 minutes. Pour into a blender and purée. Add sour cream and black pepper and blend until smooth. Taste, and adjust seasonings. Pour sauce back into saucepan and simmer over low heat.

Enchiladas

4 skinless, boneless chicken breasts

2 bay leaves

½ cup chopped fresh cilantro

½ cup chopped scallions

Salsa Verde

12 corn tortillas

1 cup grated Monterey Jack cheese

1 tablespoon chopped fresh cilantro, for garnish

Preheat oven to 400°.

Bring 1 inch of water and bay leaves to a boil in a skillet. Reduce heat to medium. Add chicken, cover and poach until cooked through, about 20 minutes, turning once. *Do not overcook.* Let cool and shred with your fingers.

In a large bowl, combine cooked chicken, cilantro and scallions with ⅓ cup salsa verde. Spoon another ⅓ cup salsa into bottom of a greased 9×13-inch baking pan.

Using tongs, dip one tortilla at a time into remaining simmering salsa. Soften tortilla in salsa about 5 seconds. Transfer tortilla onto a plate. Spoon about ¼ cup chicken filling onto center of tortilla. Roll tortilla around filling and place seam-side down in baking pan. Repeat with all tortillas and filling.

Pour remaining sauce on top of filled tortillas. Sprinkle with grated cheese. Bake until enchiladas are hot and cheese is melted, about 25 minutes. Garnish with chopped cilantro.

Fifty Cloves of Garlic and One Chicken

Makes 4 servings • Each serving: 56 grams protein • trace carbohydrate

one 3-pound chicken, cut into
  pieces

3 tablespoons pure-pressed extra
  virgin olive oil

50 peeled garlic cloves

2 tablespoons fresh lemon juice

1 teaspoon dried thyme

½ teaspoon freshly ground black
  pepper

¼ cup chicken stock (see recipe,
  page 113), or low-sodium
  canned, or water

Preheat oven to 375°. Rinse chicken under cold water and pat dry with paper towels. In a large roasting pan, heat oil over medium-high heat. When oil is hot, add chicken pieces and garlic and sauté, turning occasionally, 5 to 10 minutes.

Using a spoon, skim excess fat from pan. Add lemon juice, thyme, black pepper and stock or water. Cover tightly and bake about 35 to 45 minutes, until chicken is tender.

Garlic Chicken
with Pistachio Vegetables

Makes 4 servings • Each serving: 60 grams protein • 4 grams carbohydrate
(Nutritional information does not include Cooling Mint Sauce)

Spicy Garlic Marinade

*2 tablespoons minced garlic
cloves*

1 teaspoon red-pepper flakes

¼ cup balsamic vinegar

1 tablespoon Dijon mustard

*1 tablespoon slivered fresh basil,
or 1 teaspoon dried basil*

*¾ cup pure-pressed extra virgin
olive oil*

*freshly ground black pepper,
to taste*

Prepare marinade: In a blender or food processor, combine all ingredients and blend until smooth; or place ingredients in a jar with a tight-fitting lid and shake vigorously until well blended.

*2 pounds skinless, boneless
chicken breasts*

Spicy Garlic Marinade

*2 tablespoons pure-pressed extra
virgin olive oil*

1 medium chopped red onion

*1 red or green bell pepper, cut
into large squares*

*2 large zucchini, halved length-
wise and thickly sliced*

1 large seeded and diced tomato*

*½ cup coarsely chopped dry-
roasted pistachio nuts*

*2 tablespoons minced fresh
parsley, for garnish*

*Cooling Mint Sauce (see recipe,
page 382), (optional)*

Rinse chicken under cold water and pat dry with paper towels. Cut chicken into 1½-inch chunks and mix well with ½ cup marinade. Allow to marinate 1 to 3 hours, if possible.

Prepare barbecue or preheat broiler.

Drain chicken and reserve marinade, for basting while cooking.

In a large nonstick skillet, heat oil over medium-high heat. When oil is hot, add onion, bell pepper and zucchini and sauté until softened, about 8 minutes. Add tomatoes, pistachios and remaining marinade not already used on chicken. Cook over medium heat until heated through, about 5 minutes. Taste, and adjust seasonings. Allow to simmer over low heat while cooking chicken.

Cook chicken over hot coals *or* broil chicken on a greased rack with a tinfoil-lined baking sheet underneath. Broil 3 inches from heat source until tender, about 8 minutes. Turn and brush with reserved marinade. Slice diagonally into thin slices.

Ladle vegetable sauté on a serving platter and arrange chicken breast slices on top. Serve with Cooling Mint Sauce, if desired.

To seed tomato: Cut tomato in half and squeeze gently. Scoop out seeds with a small spoon or your fingers and dice tomato.

Ginger Chicken

Makes 4 servings • Each serving: 56 grams protein • trace carbohydrate
½ cup Basic Steamed Brown Rice: 3 grams protein • 24 grams carbohydrate

2 pounds boneless chicken breasts	1 tablespoon dry sherry
2 tablespoons pure-pressed peanut oil	1 to 2 tablespoons low-sodium tamari soy sauce, to taste
3 tablespoons peeled and finely minced fresh ginger	1 tablespoon fresh lime juice
1 thinly sliced green bell pepper	freshly ground black pepper, to taste
1 thinly sliced red bell pepper	1 tablespoon pure-pressed sesame oil
1 small thinly sliced red onion	2 tablespoons minced fresh cilantro
½ cup diced scallions	
3 minced garlic cloves	

Rinse chicken under cold water and pat dry with paper towels. Slice into thin strips. In a wok or large nonstick skillet, heat oil over medium-high heat. When oil is hot, add chicken, ginger, bell peppers, onion, scallions and garlic and sauté over medium-high heat 5 minutes. Add sherry, soy sauce, lime juice and black pepper. Mix well and cook until chicken is tender. Remove from heat. Add sesame oil and fresh cilantro and mix well. Taste, and adjust seasonings. Serve over Basic Steamed Brown Rice (see recipe, page 320).

Greek Chicken

Makes 6 servings • Each serving: 59 grams protein • 1 gram carbohydrate

3 pounds chicken pieces

¼ cup pure-pressed extra virgin
olive oil

2 minced garlic cloves

¼ cup fresh lemon juice

1 teaspoon grated lemon zest

1 tablespoon Dijon mustard

1 tablespoon dried oregano

freshly ground black pepper,
to taste

½ pound crumbled feta cheese

¾ cup diced Kalamata olives

1 tablespoon minced fresh
parsley, for garnish

Rinse chicken under cold water and pat dry with paper towels.

In a small bowl, combine olive oil, garlic, lemon juice, lemon zest, mustard, oregano and black pepper. Mix well. Arrange chicken in an ungreased 9×13-inch baking dish. Pour marinade over chicken. Marinate, refrigerated, at least 1 hour before cooking.

Preheat oven to 375°. Bake uncovered, basting occasionally, until chicken is tender, about 30 to 40 minutes. Crumble feta cheese and sprinkle olives over chicken during last 5 minutes of cooking. Remove from oven. Garnish with minced parsley.

Grilled Chicken Breasts with Artichoke Cream Sauce

Makes 4 servings • Each serving: 58 grams protein • 6 grams carbohydrate

2 pounds boneless chicken breasts

1 tablespoon Dijon mustard

1 red bell pepper or ¼ cup store-bought roasted red bell peppers

2 tablespoons pure-pressed extra virgin olive oil

1 thinly sliced red onion

1 minced garlic clove

1½ cups marinated artichoke hearts, drained and chopped

2 tablespoons slivered fresh basil, or 2 teaspoons dried basil

freshly ground black pepper, to taste

½ cup all-dairy heavy cream

¼ cup dry white wine

1 tablespoon fresh lemon juice

1½ teaspoons grated lemon zest

dash cayenne pepper

4 whole fresh basil leaves, for garnish

Rinse chicken under cold water and pat dry with paper towels. Rub chicken breasts with mustard. Cover and marinate, refrigerated 1 to 2 hours.

If using a fresh red bell pepper, roast pepper directly over a gas flame or on a rack under a preheated broiler. Using tongs, turn pepper frequently until blistered and blackened on all sides. Place pepper in a bowl with a plate on top. Let steam for 15 minutes to loosen skin. Peel off all charred skin. Discard skin along with seeds. Cut roasted flesh into thin slivers.

In a large nonstick skillet, heat oil over medium-high heat. When oil is hot, add onion and garlic and sauté until softened, about 5 minutes. Add roasted red pepper strips, artichoke hearts, basil, black pepper, cream and wine. Bring to a boil, reduce heat to low and add lemon juice, lemon zest and cayenne pepper. Simmer until sauce is thickened and reduced by ⅓, about 5 to 10 minutes, stirring occasionally. Taste, and adjust seasonings.

Prepare barbecue or preheat broiler.

Grill chicken over hot coals; *or* broil chicken on a greased rack with a tinfoil-lined baking sheet underneath. Broil 3 inches from heat source, until meat is tender, about 5 to 8 minutes per side. Spoon some sauce on each plate and arrange a grilled chicken breast on top. Garnish with whole, fresh basil leaves.

Mustard Chicken

Makes 4 servings • Each serving: 59 grams protein • 8 grams carbohydrate

2 pounds boneless chicken breasts

1½ cups fresh or dried whole-grain bread crumbs

½ cup grated Parmesan cheese

2 minced garlic cloves

2 tablespoons minced fresh herbs (rosemary, oregano, thyme, parsley)

freshly ground black pepper, to taste

3 tablespoons Dijon mustard

1 tablespoon fresh lime juice

2 tablespoons minced fresh parsley, for garnish

Preheat oven to 375°. Rinse chicken under cold water and pat dry with paper towels. In a shallow dish, combine bread crumbs, Parmesan cheese, garlic, fresh herbs and black pepper. Set aside.

Combine mustard and lime juice and spread on both sides of chicken. Coat chicken with bread crumbs, cheese and herb mixture. Arrange on a well-greased baking pan. Bake until tender, about 30 to 45 minutes. Garnish with minced parsley.

Pecan Chicken

Makes 4 servings • Each serving: 60 grams protein • 8 grams carbohydrate

6 tablespoons unsalted butter

2 tablespoons Dijon mustard

1 tablespoon fresh lime juice

1 minced garlic clove

1½ cups finely chopped raw pecans

2 tablespoons minced fresh parsley

freshly ground black pepper, to taste

2 pounds skinless, boneless chicken breasts or thighs

2 tablespoons pure-pressed extra virgin olive oil

In a small saucepan, melt butter over medium-high heat. When butter is hot and bubbly, add mustard, lime juice and garlic. Whisk together until smooth. Pour into a shallow dish. In a food processor, finely chop pecans and put into another shallow dish mixed together with minced parsley. Season to taste with black pepper.

Rinse chicken under cold water and pat dry with paper towels. Place chicken between 2 sheets of waxed paper or plastic wrap. Pound to ¼-inch thickness using a heavy mallet or back of skillet. Trim ragged edges. Dip chicken pieces in mustard-butter mixture, then in pecan mixture, thoroughly coating both sides.

In a large nonstick skillet, heat 2 tablespoons oil over medium-high heat. When oil is hot, reduce heat to medium, add chicken and cook until lightly browned and tender, about 3 minutes each side.

Pesto Chicken

Makes 6 servings • Each serving: 62 grams protein • 2 grams carbohydrate

3 pounds chicken pieces

3 tablespoons fresh lemon juice

freshly ground black pepper,
  to taste

¾ cup Basil Pesto,
  (see recipe, page 372)
  or store-bought

Preheat oven to 375°. Rinse chicken under cold water and pat dry with paper towels.

In a large shallow dish, pour lemon juice over chicken pieces. Season to taste with black pepper. Set aside for 15 minutes.

Drain chicken pieces and arrange in a greased baking dish. Spread pesto over top of chicken. Bake until tender, about 30 to 45 minutes.

Roast Chicken with Fennel and Mustard

Makes 4 servings • Each serving: 61 grams protein • 51 grams carbohydrate

one 4-pound roasting chicken

¼ cup minced fresh parsley

1 tablespoon Dijon mustard

2 minced garlic cloves

1 teaspoon red-pepper flakes

1 teaspoon crushed fennel seeds

¼ cup fresh lime juice

4 large quartered baking potatoes
(peeled, if desired)

4 carrots, cut into 1-inch
diagonal pieces

Rinse chicken under cold water, remove giblets and pat dry with paper towels. In a small bowl, combine parsley, mustard, garlic, red-pepper flakes and fennel. Mix well. Stir in lime juice to make a paste. Rub chicken with ⅔ of the marinade paste. Marinate, refrigerated and covered, 1 hour.

Preheat oven to 400°. Place chicken on a rack set in a large baking pan. Rub potatoes and carrots with remaining marinade and arrange alongside chicken on rack. Roast about 1½ hours, or until juices run clear when you pierce the thickest part of a thigh with a fork. Remove from oven and let sit 15 minutes before slicing.

Roast Chicken with Goat Cheese and Sun-Dried Tomatoes

Makes 4 servings • Each serving: 65 grams protein • 7 grams carbohydrate

one 4-pound roasting chicken

6 ounces goat cheese

½ cup sun-dried tomatoes in olive oil, drained and chopped

2 minced garlic cloves

2 tablespoons slivered fresh basil, or 2 teaspoons dried basil

2 teaspoons grated lemon zest

freshly ground black pepper, to taste

1 lemon, quartered

1 chopped onion

1 bunch coarsely chopped fresh parsley

3 tablespoons melted unsalted butter

Preheat oven to 400°. Rinse chicken under cold water, remove giblets, and pat dry with paper towels. Make a paste by combining goat cheese, sun-dried tomatoes, garlic, basil, lemon zest and black pepper. Using your fingers, gently loosen skin of breasts and legs. Spread paste between flesh and skin.

Insert lemon, onion and parsley into chicken cavity. Tie legs together with string and close opening by inserting wood skewers or toothpicks and lacing closed. Arrange chicken on a rack in a large roasting pan. Roast until chicken is tender, basting with melted butter, about 1 hour or until juices run clear when you pierce the thickest part of a thigh with a fork. Remove from oven and let rest 15 minutes before slicing.

Roast Turkey Breast

Makes 6 servings • Each serving: 93 grams protein • trace carbohydrate

*one 5-pound fresh turkey breast
 or frozen and thawed*

1 tablespoon fresh lime juice

½ tablespoon grated lime zest

*freshly ground black pepper,
 to taste*

*2 tablespoons chopped fresh
 parsley*

½ teaspoon dried thyme

½ teaspoon dried marjoram

*4 tablespoons melted unsalted
 butter*

Preheat oven to 375°. Rinse turkey under cold water and pat dry with paper towels.

In a medium bowl, using a fork, whisk lime juice, lime zest, black pepper, parsley, thyme, marjoram and melted butter. Using a pastry brush, baste marinade over entire turkey breast.

Roast turkey on a rack set in a large baking pan until tender and juices run clear when pierced with a fork, about 1 to 1½ hours. Baste occasionally. Let sit 15 minutes before slicing.

Sesame Chicken

Makes 4 servings • Each serving: 61 grams protein • 5 grams carbohydrate

2 tablespoons raw sesame seeds, for garnish

½ cup smooth organic peanut butter (no honey or sugar added)

1-inch chunk peeled and finely minced fresh ginger

3 minced garlic cloves

½ cup chicken stock (recipe, page 113), or low-sodium canned

1 tablespoon low-sodium tamari soy sauce

2 tablespoons sake, or dry sherry

1 tablespoon rice wine vinegar

1 tablespoon fresh lime juice

2 teaspoons pure-pressed sesame oil

¼ to ½ teaspoon red-pepper flakes, to taste

freshly ground black pepper, to taste

2 pounds skinless, boneless chicken breasts

⅓ cup chopped scallions, for garnish

Put sesame seeds in an ungreased skillet over medium heat. Stir seeds or shake pan almost constantly, until seeds are toasted and begin to pop, about 5 minutes. Remove from pan immediately and set aside.

In a medium bowl, combine peanut butter, ginger, garlic, chicken stock, soy sauce, sake or sherry, vinegar, lime juice, sesame oil, red-pepper flakes and black pepper until well blended.

Preheat oven to 375°.

Rinse chicken under cold water and pat dry with paper towels. Arrange chicken breasts in one layer in a 9×13-inch lightly oiled baking dish. Pour peanut mixture over chicken, turning, to coat well. Marinate 30 minutes, refrigerated, turning occasionally.

Bake until chicken is tender, approximately 30 to 40 minutes. Transfer to a serving plate. Garnish with toasted sesame seeds and chopped scallions.

Simple Lemon-Roasted Chicken

Makes 6 servings • Each serving: 56 grams protein • trace carbohydrate

one 6-pound roasting chicken

2 crushed garlic cloves

juice of 1 lemon

1 sliced lemon

6 sprigs fresh rosemary

6 sprigs fresh parsley

freshly ground black pepper,
to taste

Preheat oven to 450°.

Rinse chicken under cold water, remove giblets, and pat dry with paper towels. Rub outside of chicken with 1 crushed garlic clove and lemon juice. Fill cavity with remaining garlic clove, lemon slices, rosemary, parsley and black pepper.

Arrange chicken, breast-side up, on a rack set in a roasting pan. Reduce heat to 400°. Bake about 1 hour 15 minutes, or until tender and thigh juices run clear when pierced with a fork. Baste with pan juices.

Allow chicken to rest at room temperature 10 to 15 minutes before slicing.

Stir-Fried Chicken with Vegetables

Makes 4 servings • Each serving: 61 grams protein • 3 grams carbohydrate
½ cup Basic Steamed Brown Rice: 3 grams protein • 24 grams carbohydrate

2 pounds skinless, boneless
  chicken breasts

2 tablespoons low-sodium tamari
  soy sauce

1 tablespoon dry sherry

2 tablespoons pure-pressed
  peanut oil

1 minced garlic clove

2 teaspoons peeled and finely
  minced fresh ginger

1 thinly sliced red bell pepper

¼ pound snow peas, strings
  removed, ends trimmed

½ cup chopped dry-roasted
  peanuts, for garnish

¼ cup thinly sliced scallions,
  for garnish

Rinse chicken under cold water and pat dry with paper towels. Cut chicken into thin strips.

In a medium bowl, toss chicken strips with soy sauce and sherry. In a wok or large nonstick skillet, heat oil over medium-high heat. When oil is hot, add garlic, ginger and bell pepper. Stir-fry until softened, about 2 to 3 minutes. Add chicken strips along with marinade and snow peas and stir-fry until tender, about 3 to 5 minutes. Sprinkle peanuts and scallions on top. Serve over Basic Steamed Brown Rice (see recipe, page 320).

Tarragon Chicken

Makes 4 servings • Each serving: 57 grams protein • trace carbohydrate

2 pounds chicken pieces

freshly ground black pepper,
  to taste

2 tablespoons unsalted butter

2 diced shallots

2 cups sliced brown or white
  mushrooms

2 tablespoons pure-pressed extra
  virgin olive oil

½ cup dry white wine, or
  vermouth

1 tablespoon Dijon mustard

1 tablespoon chopped fresh
  tarragon, or 1 teaspoon dried
  tarragon

¾ cup all-dairy heavy cream

fresh tarragon or parsley sprigs,
  for garnish

Rinse chicken under cold water and pat dry with paper towels. Season chicken with black pepper.

In a large nonstick skillet, melt butter over medium-high heat. When butter is hot and bubbly, add shallots and sauté until softened, about 3 minutes. Add mushrooms and cook until softened, about 5 minutes. Remove from skillet and set aside. Wipe out skillet with a paper towel.

In same skillet, heat oil over medium-high heat. When oil is hot, add chicken and cook over medium heat until browned, about 5 minutes per side. Remove from skillet and keep warm.

Add wine or vermouth and mustard and bring to a boil, scraping bottom brown bits from pan. Whisk in tarragon and cream and simmer until sauce thickens slightly, about 3 minutes stirring occasionally. *Do not boil.*

Add chicken, shallots and mushrooms. Mix well to coat evenly with sauce. Simmer 5 to 10 minutes, until heated through and chicken is tender. Garnish serving platter with fresh tarragon or parsley sprigs.

Thai Chicken

Makes 4 servings • Each serving: 48 grams protein • 11 grams carbohydrate

2 pounds skinless, boneless chicken

Marinade

*1 cup chunky organic peanut
butter (no honey or sugar
added)*

1½ cups coconut milk

*¼ cup chicken stock (see recipe,
page 113), or vegetable stock
(see recipe, page 115), or
low-sodium canned*

*2 tablespoons low-sodium tamari
soy sauce*

¼ cup fresh lime juice

2 minced garlic cloves

*1 tablespoon peeled and finely
minced fresh ginger*

2 tablespoons chopped scallions

*3 tablespoons chopped fresh
cilantro*

2 tablespoon chopped fresh mint

2 tablespoon slivered fresh basil

*freshly ground black pepper,
to taste*

dash cayenne pepper

*twelve 8-inch bamboo skewers
soaked in water 15 minutes to
prevent burning*

Rinse chicken under cold water and pat dry with paper towels. Cut chicken into large chunks. Combine marinade ingredients in a food processor or blender and blend until smooth. Taste, and adjust seasonings. Coat chicken with ½ of marinade and marinate, refrigerated, 1 to 6 hours, if possible.

Drain and thread chicken chunks onto skewers.

Prepare barbecue or preheat broiler.

Cook chicken over hot coals; *or* broil chicken on a greased rack with a tinfoil-lined baking sheet underneath. Broil 3 inches from heat source, until chicken is tender. Turn frequently, basting until tender, about 10 to 15 minutes. Heat reserved marinade and serve on the side.

Meats

Beef

Lamb

Beef

Asian Beef Kabobs

Makes 4 servings • Each serving: 42 grams protein • trace carbohydrate
2 tablespoons Spicy Peanut Sauce: 4 grams protein • 4 grams carbohydrate

1½ pounds sirloin steak

1 tablespoon peeled and finely minced fresh ginger

2 minced garlic cloves

2 tablespoons to ¼ cup low-sodium tamari soy sauce, to taste

¼ cup pure-pressed sesame oil

½ cup finely chopped scallions

2 tablespoons minced fresh cilantro

2 tablespoons fresh lime juice

1 teaspoon grated lime zest

freshly ground black pepper

dash cayenne pepper

¼ cup dry sherry

16 whole brown or white mushrooms, stems removed

2 red or green bell peppers, cut into 1½-inch squares

1 red onion, cut into 1½-inch squares

eight 8-inch bamboo skewers soaked in water 15 minutes to prevent burning

Spicy Peanut Sauce (see recipe, page 388)

Cut beef into 1½-inch cubes and set aside. In a large shallow dish, combine ginger, garlic, soy sauce, sesame oil, scallions, cilantro, lime juice, lime zest, black pepper, cayenne pepper and sherry. Mix well. Add cubed beef, mushrooms, bell peppers and onion. Marinate, refrigerated, 1 to 2 hours.

Prepare barbecue or preheat broiler.

Thread cubed meat onto skewers, alternating with whole mushrooms, bell peppers and onion. Save marinade.

Cook skewers over hot coals, basting occasionally; *or* broil skewers on a greased rack with a tinfoil-lined baking sheet underneath, basting occasionally. Broil 3 inches from heat source, until meat is tender. Serve hot with Spicy Peanut Sauce.

Beef Stew

Makes 4 servings • Each serving: 65 grams protein • 42 grams carbohydrate

1½ pounds boneless lean beef (top round or chuck)

freshly ground black pepper, to taste

2 tablespoons pure-pressed vegetable oil

1 large chopped onion

3 minced garlic cloves

3 medium potatoes (peeled, if desired) cut into 1-inch cubes

2 carrots, cut into 1-inch chunks

2 celery stalks, cut into 1-inch chunks

1 cup thickly sliced brown or white mushrooms

28 ounces canned plum tomatoes, coarsely chopped (reserve liquid)

½ cup red wine

1 large bay leaf

1 teaspoon dried thyme

2 tablespoons chopped fresh parsley

1 cup fresh green peas or frozen and thawed

Cut beef into 1-inch cubes. Season to taste with black pepper. In a large Dutch oven or a deep saucepan, heat oil over medium-high heat. When oil is hot, add onion, garlic and beef cubes and sauté until browned on all sides. Add potatoes, carrots, celery and mushrooms and sauté 5 minutes.

Add tomatoes and their liquid, red wine, bay leaf and thyme. Bring to a boil, reduce heat to simmer and cook, covered, 2 to 3 hours, stirring occasionally. Add parsley and peas and cook 5 minutes until tender. Taste, and adjust seasonings.

California Burgers

Makes 4 servings • Each serving: 61 grams protein • trace carbohydrate
(Nutritional information does not include mayonnaise)

2 pounds ground or chopped
  sirloin, or ground turkey

½ cup diced onion sautéed in
  2 tablespoons unsalted butter

freshly ground black pepper,
  to taste

4 tablespoons goat cheese

Creamy Mayonnaise

In a large bowl, using your hands or a wooden spoon, combine ground beef, sautéed onion and black pepper. Form into 4 patties. Stuff 1 tablespoon goat cheese into center of each patty and mold beef around it.

Grill or pan-fry until cooked to your liking, turning occasionally. Serve with Creamy Mayonnaise.

Creamy Mayonnaise

Makes about 1 cup • Each 1 tablespoon serving: trace protein • trace carbohydrate

1 egg yolk*

2 tablespoons fresh lemon juice

1 tablespoon Dijon mustard

freshly ground black pepper,
  to taste

¾ cup pure-pressed canola oil

In a blender or food processor, blend egg yolk, lemon juice, mustard and black pepper until smooth. With motor running, gradually pour in oil until creamy and thickened. Store covered in the refrigerator.

---

*If you are concerned about using raw egg, choose an alternate recipe.

Chili Con Carne

Makes 4 servings • Each serving: 40 grams protein • 31 grams carbohydrate

2 tablespoons pure-pressed extra virgin olive oil

1 large diced onion

3 minced garlic cloves

1 diced green bell pepper

1 pound ground or chopped sirloin or ground turkey

1 cup beef stock (see recipe, page 112), or vegetable stock (see recipe, page 115), or low-sodium canned

14½ ounces canned diced tomatoes with their juice

2 tablespoons tomato paste

1 to 2 tablespoons chili powder, to taste

1 teaspoon ground cumin

1 teaspoon dried oregano

1 small bay leaf

freshly ground black pepper, to taste

dash cayenne pepper

15 ounces canned red kidney beans, drained and rinsed

In a large Dutch oven or skillet, heat oil over medium-high heat. When oil is hot, add onion, garlic and bell pepper and sauté until browned and softened, about 5 minutes. Add meat and brown, stirring with a wooden spoon to break up lumps.

Using a spoon, skim excess fat from pan and add remaining ingredients, except kidney beans. Bring to a boil, reduce heat and simmer, uncovered, 30 minutes, stirring occasionally. Add kidney beans the last 15 minutes of simmering. Taste, and adjust seasonings.

Classic Beef Stroganoff

Makes 4 servings • Each serving: 45 grams protein • 5 grams carbohydrate
½ cup Basic Steamed Brown Rice: 3 grams protein • 24 grams carbohydrate
½ cup Garlic Mashed Potatoes: 3 grams protein • 26 grams carbohydrate

*1½ pounds beef fillet, sirloin or
    other boneless lean beef*

freshly ground black pepper

*1½ tablespoons pure-pressed
    monounsaturated vegetable oil*

2 tablespoons unsalted butter

1 medium finely sliced onion

1 minced garlic clove

1½ tablespoons unsalted butter

1 tablespoon flour

*1 cup heated beef stock (see recipe,
    page 112), or low-sodium
    canned*

2 teaspoons Dijon mustard

1 cup whole sour cream

*1 tablespoon minced fresh
    parsley, for garnish*

Cut beef across grain into thin diagonal strips about ¼-inch thick. Season with black pepper.

In a large nonstick skillet, heat oil over medium-high heat. When oil is hot, quickly brown meat on both sides. Remove from pan and keep warm. Drain fat from pan. Add butter and melt over medium-high heat. When butter is hot and bubbly, add onion and garlic and sauté until softened, about 5 minutes. Spoon over reserved beef.

In a large saucepan, melt butter over medium-high heat. When butter is hot and bubbly, add flour and whisk until blended. Cook 2 minutes, stirring constantly. Add hot beef stock and whisk until well blended and thickened. Stir in mustard and sour cream, and heat until smooth and well mixed, about 3 minutes. Add meat and onion mixture and heat through. Taste, and adjust seasonings. Sprinkle with minced parsley. Serve over Basic Steamed Brown Rice (see recipe, page 320) or Garlic Mashed Potatoes (see recipe, page 355).

Linda Leaver's Hungarian Goulash

Makes 6 servings • Each serving: 57 grams protein • 6 grams carbohydrate
½ cup Basic Steamed Brown Rice: 3 grams protein • 24 grams carbohydrate
½ cup Garlic Mashed Potatoes: 3 grams protein • 26 grams carbohydrate

2 tablespoons pure-pressed extra virgin olive oil

2 large thinly sliced onions

3 minced garlic cloves

one 3-pound sirloin or rump roast, cubed

4 to 5 tablespoons paprika, to taste

freshly ground black pepper

3 sliced carrots

3 sliced celery stalks

28 ounces canned tomatoes, chopped (reserve liquid)

In a large heavy-bottomed Dutch oven or a deep saucepan, heat oil over medium-high heat. When oil is hot, add onion and garlic and sauté until softened, about 5 minutes. Add beef cubes, paprika and black pepper and stir well. Cover pot and simmer until juices form, about 1 hour.

Add carrots, celery, tomatoes and liquid. Simmer, covered, 5 to 6 hours, stirring occasionally. Taste, and adjust seasonings. Serve over Basic Steamed Brown Rice (see recipe, page 320) or Garlic Mashed Potatoes (see recipe, page 355).

London Broil with Aioli (Garlic Mayonnaise)

Makes 4 servings • Each serving: 56 grams protein • trace carbohydrate
(Nutritional information does not include Aioli)

one 2-pound flank steak

2 minced garlic cloves

2 tablespoons pure-pressed extra
virgin olive oil

freshly ground black pepper,
to taste

Aioli (Garlic Mayonnaise)

Preheat broiler. Rinse flank steak under cold water and pat dry with paper towels. Rub steak well on both sides with garlic, olive oil and black pepper. Place on a greased broiling pan and broil 2 inches from heat source for 5 minutes on each side or until cooked to your liking.

Cut in very thin slices on diagonal across the grain. Serve with Aioli (Garlic Mayonnaise).

Aioli (Garlic Mayonnaise)

Makes about 1¼ cups • Each 1 tablespoon serving: trace protein • trace carbohydrate

1 egg yolk*

3 minced garlic cloves

freshly ground black pepper,
to taste

½ cup pure-pressed canola oil

½ cup pure-pressed extra virgin
olive oil

2 to 3 teaspoons fresh lemon
juice, to taste

In a blender or food processor, blend egg yolks, garlic and black pepper on high until smooth. With motor running, gradually drizzle in oils until creamy and thickened. Add lemon juice and blend well. Store covered in the refrigerator.

Makes about 1¼ cups.

---

*If you are concerned about using raw egg, choose an alternate recipe.

Mama's Meat Loaf

Makes 6 servings • Each serving: 41 grams protein • 6 grams carbohydrate

*1 tablespoon pure-pressed extra
virgin olive oil*

½ cup chopped onion

2 minced garlic cloves

*2 pounds ground beef, pork
or turkey*

2 eggs

*½ cup fresh or dried whole-grain
bread crumbs*

*⅓ cup finely chopped fresh
parsley*

1 tablespoon dried oregano

1 tablespoon dried basil

*freshly ground black pepper,
to taste*

Preheat oven to 350°.

In a medium nonstick skillet, heat oil over medium-high heat. When oil is hot, add onion and garlic and sauté until softened, about 5 minutes.

In a large bowl, combine all ingredients and mix well using your hands or a wooden spoon. Lightly oil a loaf pan or 9-inch pie pan. Shape the meat into the pan.

Bake about 1½ hours. Serve with Shitake Mushroom Gravy (see recipe, page 387) or Basic Tomato Sauce (see recipe, page 378).

Middle Eastern Ground-Beef Burgers

Makes 4 servings • Each serving: 63 grams protein • 34 grams carbohydrate
Served without bun: 60 grams protein • 19 grams carbohydrate
(Nutritional information does not include Aioli)

*1½ pounds ground or chopped
sirloin*

*1 cup fresh or dried whole-grain
bread crumbs*

4 minced garlic cloves

¼ cup minced fresh parsley

1 tablespoon minced fresh mint

¼ cup whole plain yogurt

2 whole-grain hamburger buns

lettuce, tomato, onion

2 teaspoons curry powder

½ teaspoon ground turmeric

½ teaspoon ground cumin

dash cayenne pepper

*freshly ground black pepper,
to taste*

¼ cup minced scallions

1 tablespoon fresh lime juice

*Aioli (Garlic Mayonnaise)
(see recipe, page 368)*

In a large bowl, using your hands or a wooden spoon, crumble meat. Mix in remaining ingredients until well blended. Form into 4 large burgers.

Grill on a barbecue, broil or pan-fry, turning once until browned and cooked to your liking. Serve open-faced on ½ whole-grain bun with lettuce, tomato, onion and Aioli (Garlic Mayonnaise).

Savory Meatballs

Makes 4 servings • Each serving: 51 grams protein • 28 grams carbohydrate
½ cup Basic Steamed Brown Rice: 3 grams protein • 24 grams carbohydrate
½ cup Garlic Mashed Potatoes: 3 grams protein • 26 grams carbohydrate

2 tablespoons unsalted butter

1 small finely chopped onion

3 minced garlic cloves

1 pound ground beef or ground turkey

½ pound ground veal or ground turkey

1 cup whole-grain fresh or dried bread crumbs

2 tablespoons grated Parmesan cheese

freshly ground black pepper, to taste

1 beaten egg

2 tablespoons finely slivered fresh basil, or 2 teaspoons dried basil

2 tablespoons minced fresh parsley

3 tablespoons pure-pressed extra virgin olive oil

4 cups Basic Tomato Sauce (see recipe, page 378), or store-bought (no sugar added)

In a large nonstick skillet, melt butter over medium-high heat. When butter is hot and bubbly, add onion and garlic and sauté until softened, about 5 minutes. Set aside.

In a medium bowl, combine ground beef and veal or turkey, bread crumbs, sautéed onion and garlic, Parmesan cheese, black pepper, egg, basil and parsley. Mix well and shape into 1½-inch balls.

In a large nonstick skillet, heat oil over medium-high heat. When oil is hot, reduce heat to medium, add meatballs and brown on all sides. Using a spoon, skim excess fat from pan. Add tomato sauce and simmer about 20 minutes, until meatballs are tender and sauce is thickened, turning occasionally. Serve with Basic Steamed Brown Rice (see recipe, page 320) or Garlic Mashed Potatoes (see recipe, page 355).

Steak Fajitas

Makes 4 servings.
Each serving (not including salsa): 56 grams protein • 38 grams carbohydrate
(Nutritional information does not include salsa)

¼ cup fresh lime juice

2 tablespoons minced fresh
cilantro

2 tablespoons pure-pressed extra
virgin olive oil

2 minced garlic cloves

2 tablespoons chopped fresh
oregano, or 2 teaspoons dried
oregano

2 tablespoons minced red onion

2 teaspoons chili powder

1 teaspoon ground cumin

freshly ground black pepper,
to taste

dash cayenne pepper

1½ pounds top round or flank
steak, trimmed of fat

2 tablespoons pure-pressed extra
virgin olive oil

1 small fresh jalapeño pepper,
cut into thin strips; or 1 to 2
tablespoons canned diced green
chilies [wear rubber gloves to
prepare fresh jalapeño pepper]

2 thinly sliced red or green bell
peppers, cut into thin strips

1 large red onion, cut into strips

8 corn tortillas

Topping

2 sliced ripe avocados

¼ cup chopped fresh cilantro

2 cups shredded lettuce

1 cup chopped tomatoes

1 cup grated Monterey Jack
cheese

½ cup salsa (see Salsas, starting
on page 374), or store-bought
(no sugar added)

In a shallow dish, combine lime juice, cilantro, 2 tablespoons olive oil, garlic, oregano, onion, chili powder, cumin, black pepper and cayenne pepper. Mix well. Marinate steak in marinade, refrigerated, at least 1 hour or overnight, if possible.

Prepare barbecue or preheat broiler.

Grill steak over hot coals; *or* broil steak on a greased rack with a tinfoil-lined baking sheet underneath. Broil 3 inches from heat source, until meat is tender. Slice into thin strips. Set aside.

In a medium nonstick skillet, heat remaining 2 tablespoons oil over medium-high heat. When oil is hot, add jalapeño pepper, bell pepper strips and onion, and sauté until tender, about 5 minutes. Combine with sliced beef and mix well. Taste, and adjust seasonings.

Either layer corn tortillas between paper towels and microwave on high 10 to 20 seconds, *or* use tongs to heat tortillas directly over gas burner, turning once until softened and puffed up.

Serve with sliced avocado, chopped cilantro, shredded lettuce, tomatoes, cheese and salsa.

Stir-Fried Beef with Ginger Broccoli

Makes 4 servings • Each serving: 43 grams protein • 2 grams carbohydrate

2 pounds lean beef sirloin or
  flank steak

1½ tablespoons pure-pressed
  monounsaturated vegetable oil

2 teaspoons peeled and finely
  minced fresh ginger

2 minced garlic cloves

2 tablespoons minced scallions

1½ tablespoons pure-pressed
  monounsaturated vegetable oil

2 cups broccoli florets

2 cups sliced brown or white
  mushrooms

1 red bell pepper, cut into strips

½ cup beef stock (see recipe,
  page 112); or vegetable stock
  (see recipe, page 115), or
  low-sodium canned

1 tablespoon cornstarch

1 tablespoon dry sherry

1 to 2 tablespoons low-sodium
  tamari soy sauce, to taste

¼ teaspoon hot-pepper flakes

Slice beef across the grain into thin strips. Set aside.

In a wok or large nonstick skillet, heat 1½ tablespoons oil over high heat. When oil is hot, add ginger and garlic and stir-fry 30 seconds. Add scallions and beef strips and stir-fry 2 minutes. Remove from pan and set aside.

Heat remaining 1½ tablespoons oil over high heat. When oil is hot, add broccoli, mushrooms and bell pepper, and quickly stir-fry to coat with oil. Add stock and cook over high heat until boiling. Cover, reduce heat to medium and steam until vegetables are barely tender, about 5 minutes. Return beef mixture to wok or skillet.

While vegetables are steaming, mix cornstarch, sherry, soy sauce and hot-pepper flakes in a small bowl, using a fork. Stir cornstarch mixture into beef mixture and cook over medium heat until thickened and heated through. Taste, and adjust seasonings. Serve immediately.

Thai Basil Beef

Makes 4 servings • Each serving: 56 grams protein • trace carbohydrate

2 pounds beef flank steak

4 tablespoons pure-pressed
monounsaturated vegetable oil

4 minced garlic cloves

2 teaspoons peeled and finely
minced ginger

2 small, thinly sliced fresh
jalapeño peppers; or 1 to 2
tablespoons canned green
chilies, to taste [wear rubber
gloves to prepare fresh
jalapeño peppers]

1½ to 2 tablespoons low-sodium
tamari soy sauce, to taste

1 tablespoon dry sherry

¼ to ½ teaspoon red-pepper
flakes, to taste

½ cup slivered fresh basil

1 tablespoon fresh lime juice

Slice beef across the grain into thin strips. Set aside.

In a wok or large nonstick skillet, heat oil over medium-high heat.
When oil is hot, stir-fry garlic, ginger and jalapeño peppers 1 minute.
Add sliced beef and stir-fry until meat is just tender. Add soy sauce,
sherry, red-pepper flakes, basil and lime juice. Stir-fry until heated
through. Taste, and adjust seasonings.

Lamb

Grilled Lamb Chops

Makes 4 servings • Each serving: 42 grams protein • trace carbohydrate

eight 3-ounce lamb chops,
  trimmed of excess fat

4 minced garlic cloves

¼ cup pure-pressed extra virgin
  olive oil

3 tablespoons fresh lemon juice

¼ cup white wine

1 teaspoon dried oregano

1 teaspoon dried rosemary

1 tablespoon minced fresh parsley

freshly ground black pepper,
  to taste

Prepare barbecue or preheat broiler.

In a large bowl, combine garlic, olive oil, lemon juice, white wine, oregano, rosemary, parsley and black pepper. Add lamb chops and marinate at least 30 minutes, turning occasionally.

Drain lamb, reserving marinade. Grill lamb over hot coals; or broil on a greased rack with a tinfoil-lined baking sheet underneath. Baste occasionally. Cook until done to your liking, about 5 to 10 minutes on each side, depending on thickness of lamb chops.

Lamb Curry

Makes 4 servings • Each serving: 47 grams protein • 9 grams carbohydrate

2 tablespoons pure-pressed
  monounsaturated vegetable oil

2 tablespoons unsalted butter

1 large chopped onion

2 minced garlic cloves

1½ pounds boneless lamb
  shoulder, cut into 1½-inch
  cubes

1 teaspoon peeled and finely
  minced fresh ginger

1 teaspoon ground turmeric

1 teaspoon ground cumin

½ teaspoon ground cardamom

¼ teaspoon cinnamon

1 teaspoon ground coriander

freshly ground black pepper,
  to taste

1 cup whole plain yogurt

2 tablespoons minced fresh
  cilantro

1 cup fresh green peas or frozen
  and thawed

1 tablespoon fresh lemon juice

In a large skillet, heat oil and butter over medium-high heat. When hot, add onion, garlic, lamb cubes, ginger, turmeric, cumin, cardamom, cinnamon, coriander and black pepper. Sauté until lamb is browned on all sides, about 8 to 10 minutes. Reduce heat to medium, add yogurt and mix well with meat. Simmer over low heat about 10 minutes, stirring occasionally, until meat is tender.

Just before serving add cilantro, green peas and lemon juice. Cook until peas are tender and heated through. Taste, and adjust seasonings.

Lamb Kabobs

Makes 4 servings • Each serving: 42 grams protein • trace carbohydrate

½ cup finely chopped onion

2 minced garlic cloves

¼ cup fresh lemon juice

1 tablespoon minced fresh
  parsley

1 tablespoon Dijon mustard

2 teaspoons dried oregano

freshly ground black pepper,
  to taste

2 tablespoons pure-pressed extra
  virgin olive oil

1½ pounds boneless lamb
  shoulder, cut into 1½-inch
  cubes

eight 8-inch bamboo skewers
  soaked in water 15 minutes
  to prevent burning

In a shallow dish, combine onion, garlic, lemon juice, parsley, mustard, oregano, black pepper and olive oil. Add lamb cubes and coat thoroughly. Marinate, refrigerated, 1 hour or longer, if possible.

Prepare barbecue or preheat broiler. Drain and thread meat onto skewers. Grill over hot coals; *or* broil skewers on a greased rack with a tinfoil-lined baking sheet underneath. Cook, turning once and basting with marinade, until done to your liking.

Moroccan Meatballs

Makes 4 servings • Each serving: 37 grams protein • 28 grams carbohydrate

1 pound ground lean lamb

*2 medium peeled, boiled and
mashed potatoes*

2 beaten eggs

½ cup chopped fresh parsley

1 tablespoon chopped fresh mint

1 teaspoon ground cumin

½ teaspoon ground cardamom

1 finely chopped onion

2 minced garlic cloves

*¼ teaspoon freshly ground
black pepper*

¼ teaspoon cayenne pepper

¼ cup flour

*3 tablespoons pure-pressed extra
virgin olive oil*

Yogurt Mint Sauce

In a large bowl, mix lamb, potatoes, eggs, parsley, mint, cumin, cardamom, onion, garlic, black pepper and cayenne pepper. Form into small patties. Flatten sides and dredge in flour.

In a large nonstick skillet, heat oil over medium-high heat. When oil is hot, add meatballs, a few at a time, sautéeing until browned, turning frequently. Repeat with remaining meatballs. Serve hot with Yogurt Mint Sauce.

Yogurt Mint Sauce

1 cup whole plain yogurt

1 teaspoon grated lime zest

*1 tablespoon finely chopped fresh
mint*

In a small bowl, using a fork, combine yogurt, lime zest and fresh mint until well blended.

Makes about 1 cup.

Rack of Lamb

Makes 4 servings • Each serving: 56 grams protein • trace carbohydrate

1 tablespoon balsamic vinegar

2 tablespoons pure-pressed extra
   virgin olive oil

1 crushed garlic clove

freshly ground black pepper,
   to taste

3 to 4 sprigs chopped fresh
   oregano, or 1 teaspoon dried
   oregano

1 baby rack of lamb (about
   3 pounds total)

In a small bowl, combine vinegar, olive oil, garlic, black pepper and oregano. Rub rack of lamb with marinade mixture and marinate at least 30 minutes.

Prepare barbecue or preheat broiler. Grill rack of lamb over hot coals, *or* broil, fat-side down, on a greased rack with a tinfoil-lined baking sheet underneath until cooked to your liking, about 5 to 10 minutes per side.

Roast Leg of Lamb with Mustard Sauce

Makes 4 servings • Each serving: 44 grams protein • trace carbohydrate

one 3-pound leg of lamb

2 crushed garlic cloves

1 tablespoon fresh lemon juice

2 teaspoons dried rosemary

freshly ground black pepper,
    to taste

¼ cup pure-pressed extra virgin
    olive oil

Mustard Sauce

Preheat oven to 350°. Rub lamb with garlic cloves. Combine lemon juice, rosemary, black pepper and olive oil. Rub well over whole leg of lamb.

Place lamb on a greased rack set in a roasting pan and roast, uncovered, 1 to 1½ hours, basting occasionally with pan juices, until cooked to your liking. Allow lamb to sit 15 minutes before carving. Serve with Mustard Sauce.

Mustard Sauce

1 egg yolk*

1 teaspoon red wine vinegar

dash white pepper

½ tablespoon fresh lemon juice

1 minced garlic clove

1½ tablespoons Dijon mustard

½ cup pure-pressed canola oil

In a blender or food processor, blend all ingredients except oil. With motor running, drizzle in oil until sauce is smooth. Taste, and adjust seasonings.

Makes about ¾ cup.

---

*If you are concerned about using raw egg, choose an alternate recipe.

Liver

All-American Liver and Onions

Makes 4 servings • Each serving: 28 grams protein • 1 gram carbohydrate

2 tablespoons unsalted butter

1 large thinly sliced onion

1 pound calf's liver

2 tablespoons flour

2 tablespoons unsalted butter

1 teaspoon dried rosemary

1 tablespoon fresh lemon juice

freshly ground black pepper, to taste

In a large nonstick skillet, melt 2 tablespoons butter over medium-high heat. When butter is hot and bubbly, add onion and sauté until softened, about 5 minutes. Remove from pan and set aside.

Rinse calf's liver under cold water and pat dry with paper towels. Dredge lightly in flour. In the same skillet, melt remaining 2 tablespoons butter over medium heat. When butter is hot and bubbly, add liver and cook about 2 to 3 minutes, turning once, until browned on outside and pink on inside. *Do not overcook, or liver will be tough.* Add sautéed onion to pan and cook until just heated through. Sprinkle with rosemary, lemon juice and black pepper.

Pork

Ann Davis's Pigs-in-a-Blanket
(Stuffed Cabbage Rolls)

Makes 8 servings • Each serving: 30 grams protein • 10 grams carbohydrate

2 pounds ground pork, or
  mixture of pork and beef

1 cup cooked brown rice

1 large lightly beaten egg

1 teaspoon paprika

1 small minced onion

2 minced garlic cloves

freshly ground black pepper,
  to taste

1 large head green cabbage

16 ounces rinsed sauerkraut

toothpicks

3 cups Basic Tomato Sauce
  (see recipe, page 378), or
  store-bought (no sugar added)

In a large bowl, combine all ingredients except cabbage, sauerkraut and tomato sauce. Mix well using a fork or your hands.

Using a sharp knife, remove core of cabbage. Bring a large pot of water to a boil and add cabbage. As leaves become transparent, remove from water and cut out lower portion of large vein. Rinse under cold water and drain well.

Place ⅓ cup meat mixture in center of each leaf, fold sides over and roll up. Secure with a toothpick. Repeat until all of filling is used up. Pour rinsed sauerkraut into a 10-quart heavy-bottomed soup pot or Dutch oven. Place stuffed leaves on bed of sauerkraut. Add water to about 2 inches below filled leaves. Add tomato sauce. Cook on low heat for two hours, carefully stirring occasionally.

Barbecued Spareribs

Makes 4 servings • Each serving: 57 grams protein • 6 grams carbohydrate

Barbecue Sauce

2 tablespoons pure-pressed extra
   virgin olive oil

½ cup chopped onion

4 minced garlic cloves

½ cup tomato paste

1 cup water

¼ cup red wine vinegar

2 tablespoons Dijon mustard

½ teaspoon celery seeds

1 teaspoon dried thyme

1 teaspoon chili powder

1 teaspoon fresh lemon juice

freshly ground black pepper,
   to taste

dash cayenne pepper

3 pounds baby back ribs

In a medium saucepan, heat oil over medium-high heat. When oil is hot, add onion and garlic and sauté until softened, about 5 minutes. Add tomato paste and water and mix well. Add vinegar, mustard, celery seeds, thyme, chili powder, lemon juice, black pepper and cayenne pepper. Bring to a boil. Reduce heat to low and simmer about 20 minutes. Taste, and adjust seasonings.

Brush sauce over spareribs. Marinate in the refrigerator at least 1 hour or, preferably, overnight.

Prepare barbecue or preheat oven to 375°.

Barbecue over hot coals or roast on a greased rack with a tinfoil-lined baking sheet underneath. Cook until tender, basting and turning frequently, until cooked to your liking, about 15 to 20 minutes.

Kielbasa with Sauerkraut

Makes 4 servings • Each serving: 16 grams protein • trace carbohydrate

1 pound kielbasa
16 ounces sauerkraut, rinsed and
drained

½ cup water

Heat a Dutch oven or large nonstick skillet over medium-high heat. When hot, add kielbasa and sauté over medium heat until well browned on all sides. Add sauerkraut and water and bring to a boil. Reduce heat to low. Cover and simmer until sauerkraut has mellowed in flavor, to your liking, about 1 hour.

Pork Chops with Mustard Cream Sauce

Makes 4 servings • Each serving: 58 grams protein • 2 grams carbohydrate

2 tablespoons unsalted butter

1 large thinly sliced onion

2 minced garlic cloves

2 tablespoons pure-pressed extra
  virgin olive oil

four 8-ounce boneless pork loin
  chops

freshly ground black pepper,
  to taste

½ cup beef stock (see recipe, page
  112), or low-sodium canned

1 tablespoon Dijon mustard

½ teaspoon dried thyme

½ cup white wine

½ cup finely chopped fresh
  parsley

½ cup whole sour cream

In a large nonstick skillet, melt butter over medium-high heat. When butter is hot and bubbly, add onion and garlic and sauté until softened, about 5 minutes. Remove from pan and set aside.

In the same skillet, heat oil over medium-high heat. When oil is hot, add pork chops and brown on both sides. Season to taste with black pepper. Pour off excess fat from pan.

In a small bowl, using a fork, mix stock with mustard, thyme, wine, parsley and sour cream. Pour over pork chops. Cover and simmer 8 to 10 minutes, basting occasionally. *Do not boil.*

Arrange pork chops on a serving platter. Spoon sauce over chops before serving.

Roast Pork Loin with Sweet Red Peppers

Makes 6 servings • Each serving: 56 grams protein • trace carbohydrate

2 tablespoons pure-pressed extra virgin olive oil

2 minced garlic cloves

1 teaspoon paprika

2 tablespoons chopped fresh chives or scallions

freshly ground black pepper, to taste

3-pound boneless pork loin

2 tablespoons pure-pressed extra virgin olive oil

3 thinly sliced red bell peppers

1 large thinly sliced onion

8 whole garlic cloves, peeled

1 cup red wine

In a small bowl, combine 2 tablespoons olive oil, minced garlic, paprika, chives or scallions and black pepper. Rub pork loin with marinade and refrigerate 2 hours.

Preheat oven to 400°.

Place pork loin in a large roasting pan. Toss bell peppers, onion, and whole garlic cloves with remaining 2 tablespoons olive oil before arranging remaining 2 tablespoons around sides of meat. Pour wine over pork and roast 15 minutes.

Reduce oven temperature to 325°. Continue roasting pork, basting every 15 to 20 minutes, until juices run clear and meat is tender, 1 to 1½ hours, occasionally stirring vegetables and removing them from oven when tender. Remove roasting pan from oven. Allow pork to sit about 15 minutes before carving into ½-inch slices. Serve with roasted vegetables and pan juices.

Stir-Fried Pork and Vegetables

Makes 4 servings • Each serving: 29 grams protein • 3 grams carbohydrate

2 tablespoons pure-pressed monounsaturated vegetable oil

1 minced garlic clove

1 pound lean pork, cut into thin strips

freshly ground black pepper, to taste

1 diced red or green bell pepper

1 small peeled and diced jicama; or 1 cup sliced water chestnuts, rinsed and drained

2 cups stemmed snow peas

2 cups sliced brown or white mushrooms

¼ cup minced scallions

½ cup beef stock (see recipe, page 112), or vegetable stock (see recipe, page 115), or low-sodium canned, or water

2 teaspoons cornstarch

2 teaspoons low-sodium tamari soy sauce

2 tablespoons cold water

In a wok or large nonstick skillet, heat oil over high heat. When oil is hot, add garlic and pork and stir-fry until lightly browned, about 5 minutes. Season to taste with black pepper. Add bell pepper, jicama or water chestnuts, snow peas, mushrooms and scallions. Stir-fry 1 minute. Add stock or water. Bring to a boil. Reduce heat, cover and cook about 5 minutes, stirring occasionally, until vegetables and pork are tender.

Blend cornstarch, soy sauce and cold water to a paste. Add to wok, stirring to thicken. Stir until heated through. Serve immediately.

Meatless Entrées

All You Need to Know About Tofu

Tofu, an excellent source of calcium and iron, is high in protein, low in carbohydrates and is easy to digest. It is economical and can be found in most supermarkets. There are three common varieties of tofu: soft, medium and firm. Our recipes use firm tofu, because it has the highest amount of protein and the most flavor. Tofu has the reputation for being "bland," but if you follow the directions for preparing tofu you will find that it absorbs marinades well, and, when prepared with other flavorful foods, it complements and enhances many recipes.

You can find tofu packaged so that it does not need refrigeration, or in sealed containers in the refrigerated section of your market. Either way, be sure to check the expiration date. Once you have opened either type of packaging, it is best to rinse the tofu and transfer it to a jar with a tight-fitting lid. Change the water every other day. Tofu should have a sweet smell. When it is spoiled it feels slimy and has a sour odor. Even though tofu may keep for over a week or two, it is always best to eat all foods as fresh as possible.

There are two important techniques to rid tofu of its blandness and maximize its subtle flavor. First, take the tofu out of its packaging and pour off the water. Rinse in fresh water, then slice lengthwise into halves or thirds. Place the drained tofu in a shallow, flat pan. Slant the pan by propping up one edge to allow moisture to drain away. Drape a clean dishtowel over the tofu and set a heavy casserole filled with water on top to act as a weight, pressing out the excess moisture. Let the tofu drain 30 minutes.

Next, marinate the tofu for several hours or days until it "gives up" its blandness and takes on the flavor of the marinade. Prepare a marinade of your choice or use the following basic recipe. When tofu is drained and marinated it can be grilled, baked or sautéed. Enjoy the wonderful flavor of this unique food.

Basic Marinated Tofu

Makes 6 servings • Each serving: 24 grams protein • trace carbohydrate

2 pounds firm tofu, drained, pressed and sliced crosswise into 4 slabs (for directions, see "All You Need to Know About Tofu," page 291)

½ ounce dried shitake or porcini mushrooms

1 cup hot water

2 minced garlic cloves

2 teaspoons peeled and finely minced fresh ginger

½ cup rice wine vinegar

½ cup pure-pressed sesame oil

¼ cup low-sodium tamari soy sauce

2 tablespoons fresh lime juice

dash cayenne pepper

2 tablespoons minced scallions

2 tablespoons minced fresh cilantro

Prepare tofu and set aside. Immerse mushrooms in hot water and soak 15 minutes. Remove from water. Slice off and discard hard stem nubs and slice mushrooms into thin slivers. Strain the liquid that mushrooms have been soaking in through a fine sieve lined with a paper towel, and save for a future soup stock.

In a medium bowl combine slivered mushrooms, garlic, ginger, rice wine vinegar, sesame oil, soy sauce, lime juice, cayenne pepper, scallions and cilantro. Mix well with a fork. Pour over tofu. Store covered in the refrigerator. Marinate 1 hour to 2 days, turning occasionally.

Preheat oven to 375°. Remove tofu from marinade, arrange on a greased baking sheet and bake about 30 minutes, turning once. Pour marinade into a small saucepan and simmer until hot. Serve on the side with the baked tofu.

Quick and Easy Methods of Preparing Tofu

Broiling: Preheat broiler. Arrange drained and marinated tofu on a greased rack with a tinfoil-lined baking sheet underneath. Broil about 5 minutes on each side. Serve immediately.

Baking: Preheat oven to 375°. Arrange drained and marinated tofu on a greased baking sheet. Bake about 30 minutes, turning occasionally, until evenly browned. Serve immediately.

Sautéing: In a large nonstick skillet, heat 2 tablespoons pure-pressed extra virgin olive oil over medium-high heat. When oil is hot, add drained and marinated tofu and saute about 5 minutes on each side, or until evenly browned, stirring occasionally. Serve immediately.

Meatless Entrées

Black Bean and Goat Cheese Enchiladas

Makes 8 servings • Each serving: 18 grams protein • 44 grams carbohydrate

Red Sauce

*2 tablespoons pure-pressed extra
  virgin olive oil*

1 large diced onion

2 minced garlic cloves

½ teaspoon ground cumin

1 teaspoon dried oregano

28 ounces canned enchilada sauce

¼ cup tomato paste

*freshly ground black pepper,
  to taste*

In a large nonstick skillet, heat oil over medium-high heat. When oil is hot, add onion, garlic, cumin and oregano and sauté until softened, about 5 minutes. Add canned enchilada sauce, tomato paste and black pepper. Bring to a boil, reduce heat to low and simmer 15 minutes, stirring occasionally.

Enchilada Filling

1½ cups cooked, drained black
  beans

1 mango, diced

½ cup diced scallions

2 tablespoons minced fresh
  cilantro

½ cup fresh corn kernels
  or frozen and thawed

1 cup crumbled chèvre
  (goat cheese)

1½ cups whole cottage cheese

1 tablespoon fresh lime juice

2 teaspoons chili powder

freshly ground black pepper,
  to taste

12 corn tortillas

2 tablespoons minced scallions,
  for garnish

1 tablespoon minced fresh
  cilantro, for garnish

In a large bowl, using a fork, blend cooked beans, mango, scallions, cilantro, corn, chèvre (goat cheese), cottage cheese, lime juice, chili powder and black pepper. Taste, and adjust seasonings.

Preheat oven to 350°.

Pour 1 cup enchilada sauce into a 9 x 13-inch baking dish. Dip tortillas, one at a time, in simmering enchilada sauce in skillet, about 5 seconds, thoroughly coating both sides. Using tongs, transfer each tortilla to a plate. Spoon about ¼ cup filling on each tortilla, just off center. Roll tortilla around filling and place seam-side down in baking pan. Repeat with remaining tortillas.

Spread remaining sauce over filled tortillas. Bake, uncovered, 25 minutes until hot and bubbly. Sprinkle with minced scallions and cilantro.

Eggplant Parmigiana

Makes 4 servings • Each serving: 24 grams protein • 21 grams carbohydrate

1 large eggplant (peeled, if desired)
¼ cup flour
freshly ground black pepper,
  to taste
¼ cup pure-pressed extra virgin
  olive oil

2 cups Basic Tomato Sauce
  (see recipe, page 378), or
  store-bought (no sugar added)
1 teaspoon dried oregano
2 cups grated mozzarella cheese
½ cup grated Parmesan cheese

Preheat oven to 375°. Slice eggplant crosswise into ½-inch slices. Dredge slices with flour mixed with black pepper.

In a large nonstick skillet, heat 2 tablespoons of oil over medium-high heat. When oil is hot, add a few eggplant slices and sauté until softened and browned, about 5 minutes on each side. Repeat with remaining oil and eggplant slices.

Spread ½ cup of tomato sauce in a 9×13-inch baking dish. Add a single layer of eggplant slices. Top with ¾ cup of sauce and ½ teaspoon oregano. Sprinkle with 1 cup mozzarella cheese and ¼ cup Parmesan cheese. Make a second layer with the rest of the eggplant, tomato sauce, oregano, mozzarella cheese and Parmesan cheese. Bake, uncovered, until hot and bubbly, about 20 to 25 minutes.

Mushroom Zucchini Quiche with Rice Crust

Makes 6 servings • Each serving: 14 grams protein • 22 grams carbohydrate

2½ cups cooked brown rice	2 tablespoons minced scallions
2 tablespoons melted unsalted butter	freshly ground black pepper, to taste
1 beaten egg	Mushroom Zucchini Quiche Filling
1 tablespoon flour	
1 tablespoon minced fresh parsley	

Preheat oven to 350°. Lightly butter a 9-inch pie pan.

In a medium bowl, using a fork, combine cooked rice with melted butter, egg, flour, parsley, scallions and black pepper. Mix well. Gently pat into pie pan, pressing against the edges and bottom of pan with the back of a fork. Bake 20 minutes, until evenly browned.

Mushroom Zucchini Quiche Filling

2 tablespoons unsalted butter	2 tablespoons all-dairy heavy cream
1 diced small red onion	
1 pound thinly sliced zucchini	2 tablespoons grated Parmesan cheese
2 cups sliced brown or white mushrooms	
	2 tablespoons slivered fresh basil, or 1 teaspoon dried basil
1 cup whole cottage cheese, or whole ricotta cheese	
	freshly ground black pepper, to taste
3 eggs	

In a large nonstick skillet, melt butter over medium-high heat. When butter is hot and bubbly, add onion and sauté until softened, about 3 minutes. Add zucchini and mushrooms and sauté until tender, about 7 minutes. Drain well and set aside.

In a medium bowl, combine cottage cheese or ricotta cheese, eggs, cream, Parmesan cheese, basil and black pepper. Mix well, stirring with a fork. Add sautéed vegetables and pour into prepared rice crust. Bake until filling is browned and set, about 30 minutes.

Mushrooms, Snow Peas and Tofu Stir-Fry

Makes 4 servings • Each serving: 33 grams protein • 13 grams carbohydrate
½ cup Basic Steamed Brown Rice: 3 grams protein • 24 grams carbohydrate

1 cup raw cashew nuts, for topping

2 tablespoons pure-pressed peanut oil

1½ pounds firm tofu, drained, pressed and cut into ½-inch cubes (for directions, see "All You Need to Know About Tofu," page 291)

2 tablespoons low-sodium tamari soy sauce

1 tablespoon pure-pressed peanut oil

1 medium red onion, halved lengthwise and sliced in thin slivers

2 cups sliced brown or white mushrooms

2 minced garlic cloves

1 tablespoon peeled and finely minced fresh ginger

½ pound snow peas, strings removed

1 tablespoon pure-pressed sesame oil

Put cashews in an ungreased skillet over medium-high heat. Stir nuts or shake pan almost constantly until cashews are evenly browned and toasted. Remove from pan immediately and set aside.

In a wok or large nonstick skillet, heat 2 tablespoons peanut oil over high heat. When oil is hot, add tofu cubes and soy sauce and stir-fry until golden brown, stirring often. Remove from wok or skillet and set aside. Heat remaining 1 tablespoon peanut oil in wok or skillet over high heat. Add onion and stir-fry 2 minutes. Add mushrooms, garlic and ginger and stir-fry 3 minutes. Add snow peas and cooked tofu and cook until snow peas turn bright green, about 1 minute. Drizzle with sesame oil and sprinkle with toasted cashew nuts. Serve over Basic Steamed Brown Rice (see recipe, page 320).

Ricotta-Stuffed Bell Peppers

Makes 4 servings • Each serving: 24 grams protein • 11 grams carbohydrate

4 bell peppers, cut in half
  lengthwise

1½ pounds whole ricotta cheese

2 eggs

½ cup chopped Kalamata olives

1 cup chopped raw walnuts

½ cup minced fresh parsley

2 tablespoons slivered fresh basil,
  or 2 teaspoons dried basil

1 tablespoon grated lemon zest

freshly ground black pepper,
  to taste

⅔ cup grated Parmesan cheese

Preheat oven to 350°. Cut bell peppers in half and remove seeds. In a large skillet, bring 2 cups water to a boil. Add bell peppers, reduce heat to low and simmer until just tender, about 8 to 10 minutes. Remove from pan, drain and set aside.

In a medium bowl, combine ricotta cheese, eggs, olives, walnuts, parsley, basil, lemon zest and black pepper. Mix well with a fork. Mound into pepper halves. Sprinkle with Parmesan cheese. Place in an ovenproof baking dish and add water to ¼-inch depth in pan to prevent burning. Bake until heated through, about 20 to 30 minutes. Place under broiler briefly to brown top.

Grain, Legume and Rice Side Dishes

Barley

Couscous

Kasha

Legumes

Barley

Barley and Mushroom Casserole

Makes about 4½ cups • Each ⅓ cup serving: 5 grams protein • 21 grams carbohydrate

3 tablespoons unsalted butter

1 small chopped onion

2 cups sliced brown or white
   mushrooms

1 cup pearl barley, rinsed and
   drained

3 cups chicken stock (see recipe,
   page 113), or low-sodium
   canned, or water

freshly ground black pepper,
   to taste

In a large saucepan with a tight-fitting lid, melt butter over medium-high heat. When butter is hot and bubbly, add onion and sauté until softened, about 5 minutes. Add mushrooms and barley and sauté 5 minutes. Add stock or water, bring to a boil, cover and reduce heat to low. Simmer about 60 to 70 minutes until all liquid has been absorbed and barley is tender. Season to taste with black pepper.

Couscous

Basic Couscous

Makes about 2½ cups • Each ⅓ cup serving: 2 grams protein • 14 grams carbohydrate

1 cup chicken stock (see recipe, page 113), or low-sodium canned, or water

1 tablespoon unsalted butter
1 cup couscous

In a medium saucepan, bring stock or water and butter to a boil over medium-high heat. In another saucepan, with a tight-fitting lid, pour hot stock over dry couscous. Stir one time, cover and remove from heat. Let stand 10 minutes until all liquid has been absorbed. Fluff with a fork. Serve immediately.

Moroccan Couscous

Makes about 3¼ cups • Each ⅓ cup serving: 2 grams protein • 14 grams carbohydrate

*1 tablespoon pure-pressed extra
  virgin olive oil*

½ diced small onion

½ diced red bell pepper

1 minced garlic clove

1 cup couscous

1 teaspoon curry powder

*1 cup chicken stock (see recipe,
  page 113), or low-sodium
  canned, or water*

1 tablespoon unsalted butter

*½ cup fresh green peas or frozen
  and thawed*

*1 to 2 teaspoons fresh lemon or
  lime juice*

*freshly ground black pepper,
  to taste*

dash cayenne pepper

In a medium nonstick saucepan, heat oil over medium-high heat. When oil is hot, add onion, bell pepper and garlic. Sauté until softened, about 5 minutes. Add couscous and curry powder and sauté 1 minute.

In a separate medium saucepan, bring stock, butter, peas, lemon or lime juice, black pepper and cayenne pepper to a boil. Pour hot liquid over couscous, stir once, cover and let sit undisturbed 10 to 15 minutes, until all liquid is absorbed. Fluff with a fork before serving. Taste, and adjust seasonings.

Kasha

Basic Kasha

Makes about 3¾ cups • Each ⅓ cup serving: 4 grams protein • 13 grams carbohydrate

1½ cups kasha

1 beaten egg

*3 cups boiling chicken stock
(see recipe, page 113),* or
low-sodium canned, or *water*

In a medium saucepan, stir kasha and egg over medium heat until kasha has absorbed all egg, and grains are separate and dry-looking, about 3 minutes.

Add boiling stock or water. Cover and simmer over low heat until all liquid is absorbed, about 10 to 12 minutes. Remove from heat and let stand, covered, 5 minutes before fluffing with a fork.

Mushroom Kasha Pilaf

Makes about 6¾ cups • Each ⅓ cup serving: 4 grams protein • 16 grams carbohydrate

½ cup chopped raw almonds

2 tablespoons unsalted butter

1 medium diced red onion

2 minced garlic cloves

3 cups sliced brown or white
  mushrooms

1½ cups kasha

1 beaten egg

3 cups boiling chicken stock
  (*see recipe, page 113*), or
  low-sodium canned, or water

2 teaspoons low-sodium tamari
  soy sauce

2 tablespoons minced fresh
  parsley

1 cup fresh green peas steamed,
  or *frozen and thawed*

dash cayenne pepper

Put almonds in an ungreased skillet over medium-high heat. Stir or shake pan almost constantly until almonds are evenly browned and toasted. Remove from pan immediately and set aside.

In a large nonstick skillet, melt butter over medium-high heat. When butter is hot and bubbly, add onion and garlic, and sauté until softened, about 5 minutes. Add mushrooms and sauté until tender, about 5 minutes. Set aside.

Mix kasha with beaten egg and pour into a medium saucepan. Cook over medium heat, stirring constantly, until egg is absorbed and grains are separate and dry-looking, about 3 minutes.

Add mushroom-and-onion mixture, stock and soy sauce to kasha mixture. Return to a boil. Reduce heat to low. Cover and simmer until all water is absorbed, about 10 to 12 minutes. Remove from heat and let stand, covered, 5 minutes. Fluff with a fork while adding parsley, peas, chopped almonds and cayenne pepper. Taste, and adjust seasonings.

Legumes

Indian Lentil Dal

Makes about 2⅓ cups • Each ⅓ cup serving: 7 grams protein • 13 grams carbohydrate

1 cup lentils, picked over and rinsed

3 cups chicken stock (see recipe, page 113), or low-sodium canned, or water

2 tablespoons unsalted butter

2 tablespoons peeled and finely minced fresh ginger

½ teaspoon ground cardamom

½ teaspoon ground cumin

½ teaspoon ground turmeric

½ teaspoon red-pepper flakes

2 tablespoons minced fresh cilantro

1 to 2 tablespoons fresh lemon or lime juice, to taste

In a medium saucepan, bring lentils and stock or water to a boil over medium-high heat. Reduce heat to low and simmer, covered, about 30 minutes or until lentils are tender, stirring occasionally.

In a small nonstick skillet, melt butter over medium-high heat. When butter is hot and bubbly, add ginger, cardamom, cumin, turmeric and red-pepper flakes. Sauté until spices are well-coated with butter, about 3 minutes. Add spices, cilantro and lemon juice to cooked lentils. Simmer 10 minutes over low heat. Taste, and adjust seasonings.

Mexican-Style Beans

Makes about 5½ cups • Each ⅓ cup serving: 5 grams protein • 15 grams carbohydrate

2 tablespoons pure-pressed
   extra virgin oil

½ cup chopped onion

2 minced garlic cloves

1 diced green or red bell pepper

1 small diced fresh jalapeño
   pepper; or 1 to 2 tablespoons
   canned diced green chilies, to
   taste [wear rubber gloves to
   prepare fresh jalapeño pepper]

2 teaspoons ground cumin

2 teaspoons dried oregano

1 tablespoon minced fresh cilantro

4 cups cooked and drained black
   beans or pinto beans

1 cup Basic Tomato Sauce or
   Enchilada Sauce (see recipes,
   pages 378 and 383), or
   store-bought (no sugar added)

freshly ground black pepper,
   to taste

Topping

1 tablespoon whole sour cream

1 tablespoon grated Monterey
   Jack cheese

In a large nonstick skillet, heat oil over medium-high heat. When oil is hot, add onion, garlic, bell pepper, jalapeño pepper, cumin, oregano and cilantro, and sauté until vegetables are softened and nearly tender, about 8 minutes.

Add drained beans, enchilada sauce or tomato sauce and black pepper and stir well. Bring to a boil, reduce heat to medium and cook, stirring occasionally, about 10 minutes. Taste, and adjust seasonings. Serve with a tablespoon each of sour cream and grated cheese.

Middle Eastern Lentils with Vegetables

Makes about 6¼ cups • Each ⅓ cup serving: 6 grams protein • 13 grams carbohydrate

1½ cups dried lentils, picked over
   and rinsed

3 cups water

2 tablespoons pure-pressed extra
   virgin olive oil

1 medium chopped onion

2 minced garlic cloves

1 diced bell pepper

2 chopped celery stalks

2 diced carrots

1 medium zucchini, cut into
   ¼-inch half rounds

1 bay leaf

1 teaspoon ground cumin

1 teaspoon dried oregano

2 tablespoons minced fresh parsley

freshly ground black pepper,
   to taste

1 to 2 tablespoons fresh lemon
   juice

Rinse and drain lentils. In a Dutch oven or deep saucepan, cover lentils with water and bring to a boil. Reduce heat, cover and cook until lentils are almost tender, about 20 minutes.

While lentils are cooking, heat oil in a large nonstick skillet over medium-high heat. When oil is hot, add onion, garlic and bell pepper and sauté until softened, about 5 minutes. Add celery, carrots, zucchini, bay leaf, cumin, oregano, parsley and black pepper, and sauté 5 more minutes. Add vegetable mixture to lentils and mix well.

Cover and cook until lentils and vegetables are tender, about 15 minutes, adding more water to pot if needed. Add lemon juice. Taste, and adjust seasonings.

Millet

Basic Millet

Makes about 3½ cups • Each ⅓ cup serving: 3 grams protein • 20 grams carbohydrate

1 tablespoon unsalted butter

*1 cup millet, rinsed and
drained*

*3 cups boiling vegetable stock
(see recipe, page 115), or
low-sodium canned, or water*

In a medium saucepan, melt butter over medium-high heat. When butter is hot and bubbly, add millet and cook over medium heat, stirring until lightly browned, about 2 minutes.

Add boiling stock or water. Return to a boil, cover, reduce heat to low and simmer about 30 minutes or until all liquid has been absorbed. Remove from heat and let stand 5 minutes before fluffing with a fork.

Curried Millet

Makes about 4½ cups • Each ⅓ cup serving: 4 grams protein • 21 grams carbohydrate

2 tablespoons unsalted butter

1 cup millet, rinsed and drained

1 diced small onion

2 minced garlic cloves

2 teaspoons peeled and finely minced fresh ginger

1 teaspoon curry powder

1 teaspoon ground cumin

1 teaspoon ground coriander

1 teaspoon ground turmeric

dash cayenne pepper

3 cups chicken stock (see recipe, page 113), or low-sodium canned, or water

1 cup fresh green peas steamed, or frozen and thawed

1 tablespoon fresh lime juice

In a medium saucepan, melt butter over medium-high heat. When butter is hot and bubbly, add millet, onion, garlic, ginger, curry powder, cumin, coriander, turmeric and cayenne pepper. Sauté until well mixed and onion is softened, about 5 minutes.

Add stock or water. Bring to a boil. Reduce heat to low, cover and simmer until all liquid is absorbed, about 30 minutes. Remove from heat and let stand 5 minutes. Stir in peas and lime juice while fluffing with a fork.

Polenta

Basic Polenta

Makes about 3⅓ cups • Each ⅓ cup serving: 9 grams protein • 53 grams carbohydrate

4 cups chicken stock (see recipe, page 113), or low-sodium canned, or water

1 cup polenta

⅓ cup grated Parmesan cheese

3 tablespoons unsalted butter

In a large saucepan, bring stock or water to a boil. Slowly drizzle in polenta in a steady stream, stirring constantly. Reduce heat to medium-low and continue cooking, stirring frequently, until mixture thickens, about 15 to 20 minutes. Stir in Parmesan cheese and butter and serve immediately.

Polenta and Mushrooms

Makes about 4⅓ cups • Each ⅓ cup serving: 8 grams protein • 53 grams carbohydrate

2 tablespoons unsalted butter

1 cup diced onion

2 cups sliced brown or white
   mushrooms

freshly ground black pepper,
   to taste

4 cups chicken stock (see recipe,
   page 113), or low-sodium
   canned, or water

1 cup polenta

⅓ cup grated Parmesan cheese

In a large nonstick skillet, melt butter over medium-high heat. When butter is hot and bubbly, add onion and sauté until softened, about 5 minutes. Add mushrooms and sauté until tender, about 5 minutes. Season to taste with black pepper. Set aside.

In a deep saucepan, bring stock or water to a boil. Slowly sprinkle in polenta, whisking constantly to avoid lumps. Cook over medium heat, stirring, until mixture thickens and bubbles, about 15 to 20 minutes. Add onion-and-mushroom mixture and Parmesan cheese and mix well.

Polenta Variations

Grilled Polenta: Prepare Basic Polenta (see recipe, page 315). Pour cooked polenta into a greased 9×9-inch pan and spread evenly across pan. Cool until hardened. Remove from pan and cut into squares or triangles. Place on a greased baking sheet and broil until browned and crisp on both sides. Brush with compound butter before serving (see "Compound Butters," page 366).

Makes about 3⅓ cups • Each ⅓ cup serving: 8 grams protein • 53 grams carbohydrate

Polenta with Fresh Basil and Ricotta Cheese: Prepare Basic Polenta (see recipe, page 315). Add 2 tablespoons slivered fresh basil and 1 cup whole ricotta cheese as mixture thickens.

Makes about 4⅓ cups • Each ⅓ cup serving: 10 grams protein • 54 grams carbohydrate

Polenta with Gorgonzola Cheese: Prepare Basic Polenta (see recipe, page 315), substituting ½ cup crumbled Gorgonzola cheese for the Parmesan cheese, and adding ¼ cup slivered fresh basil, or 2 teaspoons dried basil.

Makes about 3½ cups • Each ⅓ cup serving: 10 grams protein • 53 grams carbohydrate

Polenta with Sun-Dried Tomato Pesto: Prepare Basic Polenta, (see recipe, page 315), adding ½ cup Sun-Dried Tomato Pesto (see recipe, page 373).

Makes about 3¾ cups • Each ⅓ cup serving: 9 grams protein • 54 grams carbohydrate

Quinoa

Quinoa (pronounced KEEN-WAA) is a grain high in thiamin, iron, vitamin B₆ and phosphorus. It was a primary food of Native Americans over five thousand years ago and a staple of the Inca civilization.

Basic Quinoa

Makes about 3 cups • Each ⅓ cup serving: 3 grams protein • 13 grams carbohydrate

2 cups chicken stock (see recipe, page 113); or vegetable stock (see recipe, page 115), or low-sodium canned, or water

1 cup rinsed and drained quinoa

In a medium saucepan with a tight-fitting lid, bring stock or water to a boil. Add quinoa and return to a boil. Cover, reduce heat to low and simmer 15 minutes until all liquid has been absorbed. Remove from heat and let sit, covered and undisturbed, for 10 minutes. Fluff with a fork before serving.

Quinoa with Spinach and Feta Cheese

Makes about 5¾ cups • Each ⅓ cup serving: 5 grams protein • 14 grams carbohydrate

2 cups chicken stock (see recipe, page 113), or vegetable stock (see recipe, page 115), or low-sodium canned, or water

1 cup quinoa, rinsed and drained

1 bunch spinach equal to about 1 cup cooked spinach, well drained and chopped; or 8-ounces packaged frozen spinach, thawed, drained and chopped

2 tablespoons pure-pressed extra virgin olive oil

2 minced garlic cloves

½ cup diced onion

1 cup chopped tomatoes

¼ cup slivered fresh basil, or 2 teaspoons dried basil

1 teaspoon grated lemon zest

½ cup crumbled feta cheese

freshly ground black pepper, to taste

In a medium saucepan, with a tight-fitting lid, bring stock or water to a boil. Add quinoa and return to a boil. Cover, reduce heat to low and simmer 15 minutes until all liquid has been absorbed. Remove from heat and let sit, covered and undisturbed, 10 minutes. Set aside.

Wash fresh spinach well, removing stems. With water still clinging to leaves, place in a medium heavy saucepan with a tight-fitting lid. Turn heat to medium-high and steam until leaves are wilted, about 2 to 3 minutes. Drain in a colander, pressing out all liquid with the back of a wooden spoon. Chop and set aside.

In a large nonstick skillet, heat oil over medium-high heat. When oil is hot, add garlic and onion and sauté until softened, about 5 minutes. Add tomatoes and cook 5 minutes. Add spinach, basil, prepared quinoa, lemon zest, feta cheese and black pepper. Mix well and cook until heated through. Taste, and adjust seasonings.

Rice

Basic Steamed Brown Rice

Makes about 3 cups • Each ⅓ cup serving: 3 grams protein • 15 grams carbohydrate

1 tablespoon unsalted butter

1 cup long-grain brown rice, rinsed and drained

2 cups chicken stock (see recipe, page 113), or *low-sodium canned,* or *water*

In a medium saucepan with a tight-fitting lid, melt butter over medium-high heat. When butter is hot and bubbly, add drained rice and sauté until grains are dried and separate. Add stock or water and bring to a boil. Cover, reduce heat to low and simmer undisturbed about 45 to 50 minutes, until all the liquid is absorbed. Remove pan from heat and let sit, covered, 10 minutes. Fluff rice with a fork and serve.

Brown Rice Pilaf

Makes about 5 cups • Each ⅓ cup serving: 5 grams protein • 24 grams carbohydrate

½ cup long-grain brown rice,
   rinsed and drained

¼ cup wild rice, rinsed and
   drained

¼ cup wheat berries, rinsed and
   drained

2 cups chicken stock (see recipe,
   page 113), or low-sodium
   canned, or water

2 tablespoons pure-pressed extra
   virgin olive oil

1 small diced onion

1 minced garlic clove

2 diced celery stalks

1 diced red or green bell pepper

1 teaspoon ground cumin

1 teaspoon chili powder

1 teaspoon dried oregano

1 cup sliced brown or white
   mushrooms

freshly ground black pepper,
   to taste

½ cup fresh green peas or frozen
   and thawed

In a large saucepan with a tight-fitting lid, bring brown rice, wild rice, wheat berries and stock to a boil. Cover, reduce heat to low and simmer until all liquid is absorbed, about 45 to 50 minutes. Remove from heat and let sit, covered and undisturbed, for 10 minutes.

In a large nonstick skillet, heat oil over medium-high heat. When oil is hot, add onion, garlic, celery, bell pepper, cumin, chili powder and oregano, and sauté until softened, about 6 minutes, stirring occasionally. Add mushrooms and black pepper and sauté 5 minutes. Stir in peas and cook until heated through.

Combine sautéed vegetables with cooked grains. Mix well, stirring with a fork or wooden spoon. Taste, and adjust seasonings.

Brown Rice with Mushrooms

Makes about 6 cups • Each ⅓ cup serving: 4 grams protein • 16 grams carbohydrate

½ cup sliced raw almonds,
  for garnish

2 tablespoons unsalted butter

2 minced garlic cloves

1½ cups long-grain brown rice,
  rinsed and drained

3 cups thinly sliced brown or
  white mushrooms

1 tablespoon low-sodium tamari
  soy sauce

freshly ground black pepper,
  to taste

3 cups chicken stock (see recipe,
  page 113), or low-sodium
  canned, or water

2 tablespoons minced fresh
  parsley, for garnish

Put almonds in an ungreased skillet over medium-high heat. Stir nuts or shake pan almost constantly until almonds are evenly browned and toasted. Remove from pan immediately and set aside.

Melt butter over medium-high heat in a saucepan with a tight-fitting lid. When butter is hot and bubbly, add garlic and rice and sauté about 3 minutes. Add mushrooms, soy sauce and black pepper and sauté 3 minutes. Add stock or water and bring to a boil. Cover tightly, reduce heat to low and simmer 45 minutes. Remove from heat and let sit, covered and undisturbed, for 10 minutes. Remove lid and fluff rice with a fork. Taste, and adjust seasonings. Spoon into a serving bowl and sprinkle with almonds and parsley.

Greek Rice

Makes about 6 cups • Each ⅓ cup serving: 4 grams protein • 15 grams carbohydrate

2 tablespoons pure-pressed extra
   virgin olive oil

1 diced small yellow onion

1 minced garlic clove

1½ cups long-grain brown rice,
   rinsed and drained

3 cups chicken stock (see recipe,
   page 113), or low-sodium
   canned, or water

3 tablespoons fresh lemon juice

2 teaspoons dried oregano

⅓ cup diced Kalamata olives

⅓ cup minced fresh parsley

freshly ground black pepper,
   to taste

½ cup crumbled feta cheese

In a medium saucepan with a tight-fitting lid, heat oil over medium-high heat. When oil is hot, add onion and garlic and sauté until softened, about 5 minutes. Add rice and sauté 2 minutes, stirring occasionally. Add stock or water. Bring to a boil. Cover and reduce heat to low. Simmer 45 to 50 minutes. Remove from heat and let sit, covered and undisturbed, for 10 minutes. Remove lid and fluff rice with a fork. Add lemon juice, oregano, Kalamata olives, parsley and black pepper. Stir in feta cheese and mix well. Taste, and adjust seasonings.

Green Onion and Lime Rice

Makes about 6 cups • Each ⅓ cup serving: 4 grams protein • 16 grams carbohydrate

¾ cup slivered raw almonds, for garnish

1½ cups long-grain brown rice, rinsed and drained

3 cups chicken stock (see recipe, page 113), or low-sodium canned, or water

¾ cup minced fresh parsley

½ cup finely slivered scallions

1 tablespoon pure-pressed sesame oil

2 tablespoons fresh lime juice

grated zest of 1 large lime

Put almonds in an ungreased skillet over medium-high heat. Stir nuts or shake pan almost constantly until almonds are evenly browned and toasted. Remove from pan immediately and set aside.

In a medium saucepan with a tight-fitting lid, bring rice and stock or water to a boil. Cover and reduce heat to low. Simmer 45 to 50 minutes. Set aside and let sit undisturbed and covered for 10 minutes. Remove lid and fluff rice with a fork. Stir in parsley, scallions, sesame oil, lime juice and lime zest. Sprinkle top with toasted almonds.

Indian Rice

Makes about 6¼ cups • Each ⅓ cup serving: 3 grams protein • 17 grams carbohydrate

¾ cup coarsely chopped raw
   cashews, for garnish

3 tablespoons unsalted butter

2 teaspoons peeled and finely
   minced fresh ginger

1 cup diced carrots

1½ cups long-grain brown rice,
   rinsed and drained

1 teaspoon ground cardamom

1 teaspoon curry powder

2 whole cinnamon sticks, broken
   into pieces

2 cups chicken stock (see recipe,
   page 113), or low-sodium
   canned, or water

1 cup coconut milk

Put cashews in an ungreased skillet over medium-high heat. Stir nuts or shake pan almost constantly, until cashews are evenly browned and toasted. Remove from pan immediately and set aside.

In a medium saucepan with a tight-fitting lid, melt butter over medium-high heat. When butter is hot and bubbly, add ginger, carrots, rice, cardamom, curry powder, and cinnamon sticks and sauté over medium heat about 5 minutes. Add stock or water and coconut milk, and bring to a boil. Lower heat, cover pot and simmer 45 to 50 minutes. Remove from heat and let sit, covered and undisturbed, for 10 minutes.

Remove lid, fluff with a fork and discard cinnamon sticks. Taste, and adjust seasonings. Transfer to a serving bowl and sprinkle with cashews.

Spinach Rice Pilaf

Makes about 8 cups • Each ⅓ cup serving: 7 grams protein • 13 grams carbohydrate

⅓ cup coarsely chopped raw
  almonds, for garnish

1 bunch spinach equal to about
  1 cup cooked spinach, well
  drained and chopped; or
  8 ounces packaged frozen
  spinach, thawed, drained
  and chopped

2 tablespoons unsalted butter

¼ cup minced red onion

1 cup long-grain brown rice,
  rinsed and drained

2 cups chicken stock (see recipe,
  page 113), or low-sodium
  canned, or water

freshly ground black pepper,
  to taste

dash cayenne pepper

Put almonds in an ungreased skillet over medium-high heat. Stir nuts or shake pan almost constantly until almonds are evenly browned and toasted. Remove from pan immediately and set aside.

Wash spinach well, removing stems. With water still clinging to leaves, place in a medium saucepan with a tight-fitting lid. Turn heat to medium-high and steam until leaves are wilted, about 2 to 3 minutes. Drain in a colander, pressing out all liquid with the back of a wooden spoon. Chop coarsely and set aside.

In a medium saucepan, melt butter over medium-high heat. When butter is hot and bubbly, add onion and sauté until softened, about 5 minutes. Add brown rice and sauté 2 minutes. Stir in stock or water and bring to a boil. Reduce heat to low and simmer 45 to 50 minutes, until all liquid is absorbed. Remove from heat and let sit, covered and undisturbed, for 10 minutes. Remove lid, fluff with a fork and stir in cooked spinach, black pepper and cayenne pepper. Mix well. Taste, and adjust seasonings. Transfer to a serving bowl and sprinkle with chopped almonds.

Tomato Vegetable Rice

Makes about 7¾ cups • Each ⅓ cup serving: 3 grams protein • 17 grams carbohydrate

2 tablespoons unsalted butter

1 tablespoon pure-pressed extra
   virgin olive oil

1 diced green bell pepper

1 medium diced red onion

2 minced garlic cloves

2 diced celery stalks

1 teaspoon ground cumin

1 teaspoon dried oregano

1½ cups long-grain brown rice,
   rinsed and drained

1½ cups diced tomatoes

3 cups chicken stock (see recipe,
   page 113), or low-sodium
   canned, or water

freshly ground black pepper,
   to taste

1 cup fresh green peas steamed,
   or frozen and thawed

2 tablespoons minced fresh
   parsley

¼ cup chopped black or green
   olives

In a medium saucepan with a tight-fitting lid, heat butter and oil over medium-high heat. When hot, add green pepper, onion, garlic, celery, cumin and oregano. Sauté until softened, about 5 minutes. Add rice and sauté until coated with butter and oil, about 2 minutes. Add tomatoes, stock or water and black pepper and stir well.

Bring to a boil. Cover tightly and reduce heat to simmer. Simmer 45 minutes, until all liquid is absorbed. Remove from heat and let sit, covered and undisturbed, for 10 minutes. Remove lid and fluff rice with a fork. Stir in peas, parsley and olives. Taste, and adjust seasonings.

Risotto

Risotto with Asparagus, Sun-Dried Tomatoes and Feta Cheese

Makes about 7 cups • Each ⅓ cup serving: 5 grams protein • 17 grams carbohydrate

3 tablespoons pure-pressed extra virgin olive oil, or oil from sun-dried tomatoes

2 minced garlic cloves

1 diced small onion

½ cup sun-dried tomatoes, drained and slivered

1½ cups long-grain brown rice, rinsed and drained

4 cups chicken stock (see recipe, page 113); or vegetable stock (see recipe, page 115), or low-sodium canned, simmering hot

½ pound asparagus, tough ends trimmed, cut into ½-inch pieces

¼ cup slivered fresh basil, or 2 teaspoons dried basil

1 cup crumbled feta cheese

1 tablespoon fresh lemon juice

2 teaspoons grated lemon zest

freshly ground black pepper, to taste

In a large saucepan, heat oil over medium-high heat. When oil is hot, add garlic and onion and sauté until softened, about 5 minutes. Add sun-dried tomatoes and brown rice. Stir gently to thoroughly coat grains with oil.

Ladle 1 cup of simmering hot stock into rice, stir well and cook over medium heat, uncovered, stirring constantly until all liquid is absorbed. Add another cup of hot stock and stir constantly until all liquid is absorbed. Continue adding one cup at a time, until all of stock has been absorbed and rice is tender. (Adding stock cup by cup will take about 20 to 30 minutes.)

Cook asparagus until just barely tender by dropping into boiling water about 3 to 6 minutes. Drain, rinse under cold water and drain again.

After all stock has been added and rice is cooked to your liking, add asparagus pieces, basil, feta cheese, lemon juice, grated lemon zest and black pepper. Taste, and adjust seasonings.

Risotto with Chicken, Mushrooms and Peas

Makes about 8 cups • Each ⅓ cup serving: 7 grams protein • 13 grams carbohydrate

3 tablespoons unsalted butter

1 small finely chopped red onion

1½ cups long-grain brown rice, rinsed and drained

4 cups chicken stock (see recipe, page 113), or low-sodium canned, simmering hot

2 cups diced raw chicken

2 cups sliced brown or white mushrooms

1 cup cooked fresh green peas or frozen and thawed

½ cup grated Parmesan cheese

1 teaspoon grated lime zest

1 teaspoon fresh lime juice

freshly ground black pepper, to taste

2 tablespoons all-dairy heavy cream

In a heavy saucepan, melt butter over medium-high heat. When butter is hot and bubbly, add onion and sauté until softened, about 5 minutes. Add brown rice and stir until grains are all well coated with butter.

Ladle 1 cup of simmering hot stock into rice, stir well, and cook over medium heat, uncovered, stirring constantly until all liquid is absorbed. Add another cup of hot stock and stir constantly until all liquid is absorbed. Repeat the same process with the next cup of stock. After the third cup of stock has been added, stir in diced chicken and sliced mushrooms. Mix well. Add remaining 1 cup of stock and continue cooking until all liquid is absorbed and chicken is tender. (Adding stock, cup by cup, will take about 20 to 30 minutes.) Add peas, Parmesan cheese, lime zest, lime juice, black pepper and cream. Cook 5 minutes longer, until peas are tender. Taste, and adjust seasonings.

Nonstarchy Vegetable Side Dishes

Baked Spinach
and Feta-Filled Tomatoes

Makes 4 side-dish servings • Each serving: 10 grams protein • 13 grams carbohydrate

2 firm large tomatoes

1 bunch spinach equal to about
   1 cup cooked spinach, well
   drained and chopped; or
   8 ounces packaged frozen
   spinach, thawed, drained
   and chopped

2 tablespoons unsalted butter

1 minced garlic clove

1 diced small red onion

½ cup crumbled feta cheese

½ cup fresh or dried whole-grain
   bread crumbs

1 tablespoon Dijon mustard

2 tablespoons slivered fresh basil,
   or 2 teaspoons dried basil

1 beaten egg

freshly ground black pepper,
   to taste

dash cayenne pepper

1 tablespoon grated Parmesan
   cheese

4 raw walnut halves, for garnish

Preheat oven to 350°. Cut tomatoes in half crosswise, scoop out pulp and seeds, leaving shell intact.

Wash spinach well, removing stems. With water still clinging to leaves, place in a medium saucepan with a tight-fitting lid. Turn heat to medium-high and steam until leaves are wilted, 2 to 3 minutes. Drain in a colander, pressing out all liquid with the back of a wooden spoon. Chop coarsely and set aside.

In a small nonstick skillet, melt butter over medium-high heat. When butter is hot and bubbly, add garlic and onion and sauté until softened, about 5 minutes. Remove from heat and set aside.

In a medium bowl, using a fork, combine prepared spinach, feta cheese, bread crumbs, mustard, basil, egg, black pepper, cayenne pepper, sautéed onion and garlic. Mix well. Mound filling into each tomato half. Sprinkle with Parmesan cheese and set on a lightly greased baking sheet. Bake 20 minutes or until filling is heated through. Garnish with a whole walnut half.

Bell Pepper Medley

Makes 4 side-dish servings • Each serving: 2 grams protein • trace carbohydrate

*3 tablespoons pure-pressed extra
virgin olive oil*

*4 bell peppers (any combination
of red, green or yellow),
cut into slivers*

1 minced garlic clove

*freshly ground black pepper,
to taste*

1 tablespoon balsamic vinegar

*2 tablespoons rinsed and drained
capers (optional)*

*2 tablespoons crumbled feta
cheese*

In a large nonstick skillet, heat oil over medium-high heat. When oil is hot, add bell peppers and garlic and sauté until softened and tender, about 10 minutes, stirring occasionally.

Remove from heat. Add black pepper, balsamic vinegar, capers and feta cheese. Toss gently. Taste and adjust seasonings. Serve at room temperature.

Broiled Eggplant

Makes 4 side-dish servings • Each serving: 7 grams protein • 4 grams carbohydrate

*1 large eggplant (peeled, if
desired)*

*¼ cup pure-pressed extra virgin
olive oil*

*1½ cups Basic Tomato Sauce or
Basil Pesto (see recipes, pages
378 and 372); or store-bought*

1 teaspoon dried oregano

1 teaspoon dried basil

*freshly ground black pepper,
to taste*

*½ cup grated Parmesan cheese,
for topping*

Preheat broiler. Slice eggplant into ½-inch-thick rounds. Lightly oil
a baking sheet.

Using a pastry brush, brush one side of eggplant rounds with olive
oil. Arrange in a single layer, olive-oil-side up, on baking sheet. Broil
about 10 minutes, about 4 inches from the heat. Turn slices and spread
tomato sauce or pesto on top side of eggplant. Sprinkle with oregano,
basil and black pepper. Broil about 5 to 10 minutes until eggplant is
tender. Sprinkle with Parmesan cheese and serve hot.

Creamed Spinach with Mushrooms

Makes 4 side-dish servings • Each serving: 3 grams protein • 3 grams carbohydrate

2 bunches spinach equal to about 2 cups cooked spinach, well drained and chopped; or 16 ounces packaged frozen spinach, thawed, drained and chopped

2 tablespoons unsalted butter

2 tablespoons chopped red onion

2 cups thinly sliced brown or white mushrooms

1 teaspoon grated lemon zest

freshly ground black pepper, to taste

2 tablespoons unsalted butter

1 tablespoon flour

1 teaspoon Dijon mustard

½ cup all-dairy heavy cream, heated until simmering

Wash spinach well, removing stems. With water still clinging to leaves, place in a medium saucepan with a tight-fitting lid. Turn heat to medium-high and cook until leaves are wilted, about 2 to 3 minutes. Drain in a colander, pressing out all liquid with the back of a wooden spoon. Chop fine and set aside.

In a large nonstick skillet, melt 2 tablespoons butter over medium-high heat. When butter is hot and bubbly, add onion and mushrooms and sauté until softened, about 5 minutes. Add lemon zest and season to taste with black pepper. Remove from pan and set aside.

Melt remaining 2 tablespoons butter in same skillet. Add flour and mustard and cook 2 minutes over medium heat, stirring constantly. Whisk in the hot cream and stir until smooth and thickened. Add chopped spinach, onion and mushrooms and stir well. Cook until heated through. Taste, and adjust seasonings.

Crustless Zucchini Quiche

Makes 8 side-dish servings • Each serving: 13 grams protein • trace carbohydrate

2 tablespoons pure-pressed extra
virgin olive oil

½ cup minced red onion

1 minced garlic clove

2 pounds zucchini, sliced into
thin rounds

4 eggs

1 cup all-dairy heavy cream

¼ cup chopped fresh parsley

2 teaspoons dried oregano

4 ounces canned diced chilies

2 cups grated Monterey Jack
cheese

freshly ground black pepper,
to taste

Preheat oven to 350°. In a large nonstick skillet, heat oil over medium-high heat. When oil is hot, add onion and garlic and sauté until softened, about 5 minutes. Add sliced zucchini and sauté 5 minutes until barely tender.

In a large bowl, using a fork, whisk eggs and cream until well blended. Stir in zucchini and onion mixture, parsley, oregano, chilies, Monterey Jack cheese and black pepper. Mix well. Spoon into a greased oven-proof casserole or 9-inch pie pan and bake about 40 minutes, or until egg custard is set in center. A knife inserted into the center of the quiche should come out clean. Let sit 10 minutes before slicing.

Curried Cauliflower

Makes 4 side-dish servings • Each serving: 4 grams protein • 3 grams carbohydrate

1 cup water

1 large head cauliflower,
separated into florets

2 tablespoons unsalted butter

2 tablespoons pure-pressed
monounsaturated vegetable oil

1 large diced onion

1 teaspoon mustard seeds

2 minced garlic cloves

2 teaspoons peeled and finely
minced fresh ginger

1 teaspoon ground coriander

1 teaspoon ground cumin

1 teaspoon ground turmeric

1 teaspoon curry powder

freshly ground black pepper,
to taste

dash cayenne pepper

1 tablespoon fresh lemon or lime
juice

1 cup whole plain yogurt

1 tablespoon chopped fresh
cilantro, for garnish

In a large saucepan, bring water to a boil. Add cauliflower florets and cook until barely tender, about 5 minutes. Drain and set aside.

In a large nonstick skillet, heat butter and oil over medium-high heat. When hot, add onion and sauté until softened, about 5 minutes. Add mustard seeds and stir until seeds begin to pop, about 1 minute.

Add garlic, ginger, coriander, cumin, turmeric, curry powder, black pepper and cayenne pepper. Stir and cook until well mixed, about 2 minutes. Reduce heat to low. Add lemon or lime juice and yogurt, and mix well. Add cooked cauliflower. Stir until well blended and evenly coated with curry spices. Taste, and adjust seasonings. Sprinkle with chopped cilantro before serving.

Green Beans in Peanut Sauce

Makes 4 side-dish servings • Each serving: 6 grams protein • 4 grams carbohydrate

1 pound fresh green beans, ends trimmed, and sliced diagonally into 1-inch pieces

3 tablespoons organic peanut butter, smooth or chunky (no honey or sugar added)

1 cup vegetable stock (see recipe, page 115), or low-sodium canned, or water

1 minced garlic clove

2 teaspoons peeled and finely minced fresh ginger

1 tablespoon lime juice

¼ teaspoon cayenne pepper

1 tablespoon low-sodium tamari soy sauce

1 tablespoon minced fresh cilantro, for garnish

Cook green beans in boiling water until just tender, about 5 minutes or more. Drain and set aside.

In a small saucepan, bring peanut butter, stock or water, garlic, ginger, lime juice, cayenne pepper and soy sauce to a boil. Reduce heat and simmer 5 minutes. Taste, and adjust seasonings.

Pour sauce over green beans. Sprinkle with cilantro and serve immediately.

Green Beans with Sesame Mayonnaise

Makes 4 side-dish servings • Each serving: 1 gram protein • 1 gram carbohydrate

1 tablespoon raw sesame seeds, for garnish

1 pound fresh green beans, ends trimmed

⅓ cup mayonnaise (made from pure-pressed oil)

2 tablespoons whole sour cream

2 teaspoons fresh lime juice

½ teaspoon pure-pressed sesame oil

freshly ground black pepper, to taste

dash cayenne pepper

Put sesame seeds in an ungreased skillet over medium-high heat. Shake pan or stir seeds almost constantly until seeds are evenly browned and toasted and begin to pop. Remove from pan immediately and set aside.

Cook green beans in boiling water until just tender, about 5 minutes or more. Drain well and arrange on a serving platter.

In a small bowl, using a fork, mix mayonnaise, sour cream, lime juice, sesame oil, black pepper and cayenne pepper until well blended. Taste, and adjust seasonings.

Pour sauce over green beans and sprinkle with sesame seeds. Serve at room temperature.

Indonesian Asparagus

Makes 4 side-dish servings • Each serving: 6 grams protein • 2 grams carbohydrate

2 tablespoons pure-pressed
  peanut oil

½ cup chopped red onion

1 teaspoon dried cardamom

½ teaspoon red-pepper flakes

2 teaspoons ground coriander

2 teaspoons peeled and finely
  minced fresh ginger

2 tablespoons creamy organic
  peanut butter (no honey or
  sugar added)

2 tablespoons fresh lime juice

1 can (14 ounces) coconut milk

1 tablespoon minced fresh
  cilantro

1 tablespoon chopped scallions

freshly ground black pepper,
  to taste

2 pounds fresh asparagus,
  tough ends trimmed, cut
  into 1½-inch pieces

In a large nonstick skillet, heat oil over medium-high heat. When oil is hot, add onion and sauté until softened, about 5 minutes. Add cardamom, red-pepper flakes, coriander, ginger, peanut butter, lime juice, coconut milk, cilantro, scallions and black pepper. Mix well. Bring to a boil, reduce heat to low and simmer 2 minutes.

Add asparagus and cook until tender, about 3 to 6 minutes. Taste, and adjust seasonings. Serve immediately.

Italian Cauliflower

Makes 4 side-dish servings • Each serving: 4 grams protein • 3 grams carbohydrate

*1 large head cauliflower,
separated into florets*

*1 cup Basic Tomato Sauce
(see recipe, page 378), or
store-bought*

*2 tablespoons rinsed and
drained capers*

¼ cup chopped green olives

*freshly ground black pepper,
to taste*

*2 tablespoons grated Parmesan
cheese, for garnish*

*1 tablespoon minced fresh
parsley, for garnish*

In a large saucepan, bring water to a boil. Add cauliflower florets and steam until barely tender, about 5 minutes. Drain and set aside.

In a medium saucepan, heat tomato sauce over medium heat until simmering hot. Add capers, green olives, cauliflower and black pepper. Cook until heated through. Taste, and adjust seasonings. Garnish with Parmesan cheese and parsley and serve immediately.

Piperade
(Bell Pepper and Tomato Stew)

Makes 6 side-dish servings • Each serving: 2 grams protein • 2 grams carbohydrate

2 tablespoons pure-pressed extra virgin olive oil

1 large onion, sliced into thin slivers

1 minced garlic clove

2 red bell peppers, cut into thin slivers

2 green bell peppers, cut into thin slivers

4 large tomatoes, peeled, seeded and chopped*

2 tablespoons slivered fresh basil, or 2 teaspoons dried basil

¼ teaspoon red-pepper flakes

freshly ground black pepper, to taste

In a large nonstick skillet, heat oil over medium-high heat. When oil is hot, add onion, garlic and bell peppers and sauté over medium heat until softened, about 5 minutes.

Add tomatoes, basil, red-pepper flakes and black pepper. Cook uncovered over medium heat, stirring occasionally, until mixture thickens and most of tomato liquid has evaporated, about 30 minutes. Taste, and adjust seasonings.

---

*To peel and seed tomatoes: Plunge tomatoes into boiling water for several seconds, then into cold water. The skins will slip off easily. Cut tomatoes in half and squeeze gently. Scoop out seeds using a small spoon or your fingers.

Ratatouille

Makes 6 side-dish servings • Each serving: 4 grams protein • 3 grams carbohydrate

3 tablespoons pure-pressed extra
   virgin olive oil

1 large chopped onion

3 minced garlic cloves

1 large eggplant, (peeled, if desired)
   cut into ½-inch cubes

1 red bell pepper, cut into ½-inch
   pieces

1 green bell pepper, cut into
   ½-inch pieces

1 large zucchini, cut into ¼-inch
   half circles

1 cup green beans, ends trimmed,
   and sliced diagonally into
   1-inch pieces

6 chopped ripe large tomatoes

2 tablespoons tomato paste

¼ cup chopped fresh parsley

¼ cup red wine

½ cup water

2 tablespoons slivered fresh basil,
   or 2 teaspoons dried basil

½ teaspoon dried thyme

½ teaspoon dried rosemary

½ teaspoon dried marjoram

1 bay leaf

1 tablespoon balsamic vinegar

finely ground black pepper,
   to taste

In a large Dutch oven or flameproof casserole, heat oil over
medium-high heat. When oil is hot, add onion and garlic and sauté
until softened, about 5 minutes.

Add eggplant and bell peppers and cook until softened, about 8
more minutes. Add zucchini, green beans, tomatoes, tomato paste,
parsley, wine, water and herbs. Mix well. Bring to a boil, reduce heat
and simmer, uncovered, 20 minutes, stirring occasionally.

Add balsamic vinegar and black pepper. Taste, and adjust seasonings. Simmer 15 more minutes. Serve hot, warm or cold.

Roasted Pepper Medley

Makes 6 side-dish servings • Each serving: trace protein • trace carbohydrate

6 assorted peppers, red, yellow,
  green and pasilla

¼ cup pure-pressed extra virgin
  olive oil

2 minced garlic cloves

2 tablespoons balsamic vinegar

1 tablespoon Dijon mustard

freshly ground black pepper,
  to taste

Roast peppers directly over a gas flame, or under preheated broiler on a broiler rack. Using tongs, turn peppers frequently until blistered and blackened on all sides. Place peppers in a bowl with a plate on top. Let steam for 15 minutes to loosen skins. Peel off all charred skin. Discard skin along with seeds. Cut roasted flesh into slivers.

In a small bowl, using a fork, mix olive oil, garlic, balsamic vinegar, mustard and black pepper until well blended. Pour over peppers and marinate at least 15 minutes before serving at room temperature.

Sautéed Mixed Squash with Cumin and Chili Powder

Makes 4 side-dish servings • Each serving: 2 grams protein • trace carbohydrate

4 small crookneck yellow squash, cut into ¼-inch rounds

4 small zucchini, cut into ¼-inch rounds

2 tablespoons pure-pressed extra virgin olive oil

2 minced garlic cloves

1 teaspoon chili powder

1 teaspoon ground cumin

1 teaspoon dried oregano

freshly ground black pepper, to taste

2 tablespoons fresh lime juice

In a medium saucepan, boil 1 cup water. Add squash and zucchini and cook until barely tender, stirring occasionally, 3 to 5 minutes. Using a slotted spoon, remove squash from pan and drain well. Set aside.

In a large nonstick skillet, heat oil over medium-high heat. When oil is hot, add garlic, chili powder, cumin, oregano and black pepper. Sauté until spices are well-coated with oil.

Add reserved squash and lime juice and toss gently until well-coated with spices and heated through. Taste, and adjust seasonings.

Sautéed Mushrooms

Makes 4 side-dish servings • Each serving: 3 grams protein • 2 grams carbohydrate

3 tablespoons unsalted butter

¼ cup chopped scallions

1 pound thickly sliced brown or
  white mushrooms

2 teaspoons low-sodium tamari
  soy sauce

2 tablespoons dry sherry

freshly ground black pepper,
  to taste

In a large nonstick skillet, melt butter over medium-high heat. When butter is hot and bubbly, add scallions and mushrooms and sauté until mushrooms are tender, about 5 minutes. Stir in soy sauce, sherry and black pepper.

Sesame Broccoli

Makes 6 side-dish servings • Each serving: 3 grams protein • trace carbohydrate

2 teaspoons raw sesame seeds,
  for garnish

2 bunches broccoli, cut into
  bite-size florets

1 tablespoon pure-pressed
  sesame oil

1 tablespoon rice wine vinegar

2 teaspoons low-sodium tamari
  soy sauce

freshly ground black pepper,
  to taste

Put sesame seeds in an ungreased skillet over medium-high heat. Stir seeds or shake pan almost constantly until seeds are evenly browned and toasted and begin to pop. Remove from pan immediately and set aside.

In a large saucepan, bring 2 cups water to a boil. Add broccoli florets and cook until barely tender, about 5 to 7 minutes. Drain and set aside.

In a small bowl, using a fork, mix sesame oil, rice wine vinegar, soy sauce and black pepper. Toss gently with steamed broccoli. Taste, and adjust seasonings. Sprinkle with sesame seeds before serving.

Sun-Dried Tomato Cooked Spinach

Makes 4 side-dish servings • Each serving: 3 grams protein • 7 grams carbohydrate

*2 bunches spinach equal to about
2 cups cooked spinach, well
drained and chopped; or
16 ounces packaged frozen
spinach, thawed, drained
and chopped*

*½ cup Sun-Dried Tomato Pesto
(see recipe, page 373), or
store-bought*

¼ cup all-dairy heavy cream

Wash spinach well, removing stems. With water still clinging to leaves, place in a medium saucepan with a tight-fitting lid. Turn heat to medium-high and steam until leaves are wilted, about 2 to 3 minutes. Drain in a colander, pressing out all liquid with the back of a wooden spoon. Chop fine and set aside.

In a food processor, blend cooked and drained spinach with tomato pesto and cream until smooth. Taste, and adjust seasonings.

Transfer to a small saucepan and gently heat through. *Do not boil.*

Vegetable Stir-Fry

Makes 4 side-dish servings • Each serving: 3 grams protein • 2 grams carbohydrate

2 tablespoons pure-pressed
  peanut oil

2 teaspoons peeled and finely
  minced fresh ginger

2 minced garlic cloves

1 cup thinly slivered carrots

1 cup thinly slivered zucchini

1 thinly sliced green or red bell
  pepper

2 cups thinly sliced brown or
  white mushrooms

1 tablespoon low-sodium tamari
  soy sauce

½ cup vegetable stock (see recipe,
  page 115), or low-sodium
  canned, or water

2 teaspoons pure-pressed sesame
  oil

1 tablespoon chopped scallions

In a wok or a large nonstick skillet, heat peanut oil over medium-high heat. When oil is hot, add ginger and garlic and stir-fry, about 30 seconds. Add carrots, zucchini and bell pepper and stir-fry 2 minutes. Add mushrooms and stir-fry 2 more minutes.

Sprinkle with soy sauce and stir-fry until well blended. Add stock or water and turn heat to high. Cover and cook about 2 minutes, or until vegetables are tender.

Sprinkle with sesame oil and chopped scallions.

Zucchini Eggplant Tomato Trio

Makes 4 side-dish servings • Each serving: 4 grams protein • 2 grams carbohydrate

2 tablespoons pure-pressed extra virgin olive oil

2 medium thinly sliced red onions

2 minced garlic cloves

4 ripe medium tomatoes

4 medium zucchini

3 small Japanese eggplant (peeled, if desired)

¼ cup pure-pressed extra virgin olive oil

freshly ground black pepper, to taste

1 tablespoon chopped fresh thyme, or 2 teaspoons dried thyme

2 tablespoons grated Parmesan cheese

Preheat oven to 350°. In a large nonstick skillet, heat oil over medium-high heat. When oil is hot, add onion and garlic, and sauté until softened, about 5 minutes. Spread onion in bottom of an 8-inch-square baking dish.

Slice tomatoes, zucchini and eggplant into thin ¼-inch slices. On top of onion, make a row of sliced zucchini down the length of baking pan. Next, make a row of eggplant, overlapping zucchini about halfway. Next, make a row of tomato slices, overlapping eggplant row by half. Continue making rows until all vegetables are used.

Drizzle olive oil over vegetables. Sprinkle with black pepper and thyme. Bake until vegetables are tender, about 30 minutes. Increase oven temperature to 475°. Sprinkle with grated Parmesan cheese and cook 5 minutes, until top is lightly browned.

Zucchini with Basil, Parmesan Cheese and Toasted Almonds

Makes 4 side-dish servings • Each serving: 2 grams protein • trace carbohydrate

2 tablespoons sliced raw almonds, for garnish

4 medium zucchini

2 tablespoons pure-pressed extra virgin olive oil

1 minced garlic clove

freshly ground black pepper, to taste

1 tablespoon slivered fresh basil, or 1 teaspoon dried basil

2 tablespoons grated Parmesan cheese

Put almonds in an ungreased skillet over medium-high heat. Stir or shake pan almost constantly, until almonds are evenly browned and toasted. Remove from pan immediately and set aside.

Trim ends of zucchini and cut lengthwise into ¼-inch-thick slices. Cut slices into 1-inch squares.

In a large nonstick skillet, heat oil over medium-high heat. When oil is hot, add garlic and zucchini and sauté until zucchini is tender, about 5 to 7 minutes. Stir frequently. Remove from heat, add black pepper, basil and Parmesan cheese. Taste, and adjust seasonings.

Transfer to a serving bowl and sprinkle with sliced almonds.

Starchy Vegetable Side Dishes

Garlic Mashed Potatoes

Makes 6 side-dish servings • Each serving: 3 grams protein • 26 grams carbohydrate

1 bulb garlic

1½ pounds russet potatoes, peeled if desired

⅓ cup all-dairy heavy cream, heated to a simmer

3 tablespoons melted unsalted butter

freshly ground black pepper, to taste

Preheat oven to 450°. With a sharp knife, slice off the top ½ inch of the garlic bulb and discard or save for another use. Drizzle the bulb with olive oil and black pepper. In a small baking dish, bake garlic until cloves pop out of their skins, about 15 minutes. Set aside. When cool, squeeze cloves out of skins and mince.

Cook potatoes in boiling water until fork-tender, about 15 to 20 minutes. Drain and return to pot. Mash with a fork or potato masher, adding heated cream, butter and roasted garlic. Season to taste with black pepper.

Jitka Gunaratna's Potato Pancakes

Makes 4 side-dish servings • Each serving: 5 grams protein • 26 grams carbohydrate

2 large russet baking potatoes

1 egg

2 to 3 minced garlic cloves

1 teaspoon marjoram

freshly ground black pepper, to taste

3 tablespoons unsalted butter

Peel and grate potatoes. Place grated potatoes in a sieve for 10 minutes to drain into a bowl. Set drained water aside to allow starch to settle to bottom of bowl.

In medium bowl, beat egg with a fork. Add drained potatoes, garlic, marjoram and black pepper. Mix well. Drain potato water from bowl and discard. Mix remaining starch, from bottom of the bowl, into potato mixture.

In a large nonstick skillet, melt butter. When butter is hot and bubbly, spoon dollops of batter into pan. Form pancakes by flattening slightly with the back of a spoon. Cook until golden brown on bottom before turning. Drain on paper towels.

Oven-Roasted Sweet Potatoes

Makes 6 side-dish servings • Each serving: 1 gram protein • 14 grams carbohydrate

1½ pounds sweet potatoes

3 tablespoons pure-pressed extra
  virgin olive oil

freshly ground black pepper,
  to taste

Preheat oven to 450°. Peel sweet potatoes and cut into 1½-inch chunks. Toss with olive oil and black pepper. Spread in a single layer on a greased baking sheet. Roast about 20 to 30 minutes, stirring occasionally, until evenly browned and tender.

Potato Gratin

Makes 6 side-dish servings • Each serving: 6 grams protein • 42 grams carbohydrate

2 tablespoons unsalted butter

2 minced garlic cloves

1 tablespoon flour

1 cup all-dairy heavy cream, heated to simmering

2¼ pounds russet potatoes (peeled, if desired) cut into ¼-inch-thick rounds

freshly ground black pepper, to taste

1 tablespoon melted unsalted butter

¼ cup fresh or dried whole-grain bread crumbs

¼ cup grated Parmesan cheese

Preheat oven to 350°. In a small nonstick skillet, melt butter over medium-high heat. When butter is hot and bubbly, add garlic and stir until softened, about 30 seconds. Add flour and cook 3 minutes, stirring constantly. Stir in heated cream and bring to a simmer, stirring occasionally, cooking until thickened, about 1-2 minutes. *Do not boil.*

Butter an oven-proof 11-inch casserole or similar size dish. Arrange potatoes in overlapping layers. Season to taste with black pepper. Pour cream mixture over top.

Bake 1 hour or longer, until potatoes are tender. Sprinkle with melted butter, bread crumbs and Parmesan cheese and place briefly under broiler until lightly browned.

Puréed Acorn Squash

Makes 4 side-dish servings • Each serving: 12 grams protein • 14 grams carbohydrate

2 acorn squash, cut in half and
   seeded

2 tablespoons unsalted butter

freshly ground black pepper,
   to taste

Preheat oven to 450°. Place squash cavity-side up in a baking pan. Add 1 inch of water to prevent burning. Dot ½ tablespoon of butter into each squash cavity. Roast in oven, uncovered, until squash is tender and lightly browned, about 30 to 40 minutes.

Scoop out squash pulp and discard skin. In a blender or food processor, purée pulp until smooth. Season to taste with black pepper.

Roasted Potatoes with Garlic and Cheese

Makes 6 side-dish servings • Each serving: 7 grams protein • 20 grams carbohydrate

2 pounds small red potatoes
   (peeled if desired)

1½ tablespoons pure-pressed
   extra virgin olive oil

freshly ground pepper, to taste

10 whole peeled garlic cloves,
   mixed with 1 teaspoon pure-
   pressed extra virgin olive oil

½ cup crumbled feta or
   Gorgonzola cheese

2 tablespoons minced fresh
   parsley

Preheat oven to 475°. Slice potatoes into quarters. In a large bowl, toss with olive oil, garlic cloves and black pepper.

Spread potatoes on a lightly greased baking sheet and roast 30 minutes, stirring occasionally. Add whole garlic cloves the last 15 minutes. Remove from oven and toss gently with feta or Gorgonzola cheese and minced parsley.

Stir-Fried Red Potatoes and Cabbage

Makes 6 side-dish servings • Each serving: 3 grams protein • 13 grams carbohydrate

2 tablespoons pure-pressed extra
  virgin olive oil

1 tablespoon unsalted butter

4 medium red potatoes,
  (peeled, if desired) diced
  into ½-inch cubes

2 teaspoons peeled and finely
  minced fresh ginger

1 teaspoon ground cumin

¼ teaspoon red-pepper flakes

1 pound finely sliced
  Napa or Savoy cabbage

freshly ground black pepper,
  to taste

In a large nonstick skillet, heat oil and butter over medium-high heat. When hot, add diced potatoes, ginger, cumin and red-pepper flakes. Sauté until potatoes are evenly browned and tender, about 15 minutes. Add cabbage and stir constantly, until tender and bright green, about 5 minutes. Season to taste with black pepper.

Stuffed Baked Potatoes

Makes 8 side-dish servings • Each side-dish serving: 9 grams protein • 35 grams carbohydrate

4 large baking potatoes	¼ cup pesto (see Pestos, starting on page 371), or store-bought
2 tablespoons pure-pressed extra virgin olive oil	½ cup crumbled feta cheese
1 small diced onion	freshly ground black pepper, to taste
1 cup chopped brown or white mushrooms	paprika, for garnish

Preheat oven to 425°. Scrub potatoes and prick with a knife in several places. Bake directly on oven rack 1 hour or until soft. Cut potatoes in half lengthwise and scoop out insides, leaving a ¼-inch-thick shell.

In a medium nonstick skillet, heat oil over medium-high heat. When oil is hot, add onion and mushrooms and sauté until softened and all mushroom liquid has been absorbed, about 6 to 8 minutes. In a large bowl, combine scooped-out potato filling, onion and mushrooms, pesto, crumbled feta cheese and black pepper.

Stuff mixture back into potato shells, mounding on top. Place on a baking sheet. Reduce oven temperature to 350° and bake until heated through, about 30 minutes. Sprinkle tops of potatoes with paprika before serving.

Chutney,
Compound Butters,
Mayonnaise, Pestos,
Salsas and Sauces

Chutney

Compound Butters

Mayonnaise

Pestos

Salsas

Sauces

Chutney

Apricot and Raisin Chutney

Makes about 1 cup • 1 tablespoon: 1 gram protein • 7 grams carbohydrate

Serve with Indian curries.

½ cup raisins   2 tablespoons fresh lime juice
½ cup dried apricots   dash cayenne pepper
½ cup boiling water

In a small bowl, soak raisins and apricots in boiling water for 15 minutes. Transfer to a blender or food processor and add lime juice and cayenne pepper. Process until well blended and smooth. Taste, and adjust seasonings. Cover and refrigerate.

Compound Butters

To prepare compound butter, let 1 stick of butter soften at room temperature. Mix in fresh herbs and seasonings. Scoop blended butter onto center of a piece of plastic wrap or waxed paper. Roll into a 6-inch log, sealing edges. Refrigerate until firm. Cut off pats of butter as needed. (The logs may also be frozen.) To serve, melt a pat of compound butter on any hot dish.

Caper Butter

Makes about ½ cup • 1 tablespoon: trace protein • trace carbohydrate

1 stick unsalted butter

2 tablespoons rinsed and drained chopped capers

2 tablespoons chopped fresh tarragon, or 2 teaspoons dried tarragon

freshly ground black pepper, to taste

Curry Butter

Makes about ½ cup • 1 tablespoon: trace protein • trace carbohydrate

1 stick unsalted butter

1 teaspoon curry powder

1 teaspoon minced fresh cilantro

1 teaspoon minced scallions

freshly ground black pepper, to taste

Fresh Basil Butter

Makes about ½ cup • 1 tablespoon: trace protein • trace carbohydrate

1 stick unsalted butter

1 tablespoon fresh lemon juice

2 tablespoons slivered fresh basil,
   or 2 teaspoons dried basil

freshly ground black pepper,
   to taste

Fresh Lemon Butter

Makes about ½ cup • 1 tablespoon: trace protein • trace carbohydrate

1 stick unsalted butter

1 tablespoon fresh lemon juice

1 teaspoon grated lemon zest

1 tablespoon minced fresh
   parsley

freshly ground black pepper,
   to taste

Garlic Cilantro Lime Butter

Makes about ½ cup • 1 tablespoon: trace protein • trace carbohydrate

1 stick unsalted butter

2 tablespoons chopped fresh
   cilantro

2 teaspoons fresh lime juice

2 minced garlic cloves

freshly ground black pepper,
   to taste

Mayonnaise

Aioli (Garlic Mayonnaise)

Makes about 1¼ cups • 1 tablespoon: trace protein • trace carbohydrate

Use as a dip, sandwich spread or sauce for fish and chicken.

*1 egg yolk**

3 minced garlic cloves

freshly ground black pepper,
to taste

½ cup pure-pressed canola oil

½ cup pure-pressed extra virgin
olive oil

2 to 3 teaspoons fresh lemon
juice, to taste

In a blender or food processor, blend egg yolk, garlic and black pepper on high until smooth. With motor running, gradually drizzle in oils until creamy and thickened. Add lemon juice and blend well. Store covered in refrigerator.

---

*If you are concerned about using raw egg, choose an alternate recipe.

Creamy Mayonnaise

Makes about 1 cup • 1 tablespoon: trace protein • trace carbohydrate

Delicious with grilled fish, chicken, meat or on sandwiches.

1 egg yolk*

2 tablespoons fresh lemon juice

1 tablespoon Dijon mustard

freshly ground black pepper, to taste

¾ cup pure-pressed canola oil

In a blender or food processor, blend egg yolk, lemon juice, mustard and black pepper until smooth. With motor running, gradually pour in oil until creamy and thickened. Store covered in refrigerator.

Curried Mayonnaise

Makes about 1¼ cups • 1 tablespoon: trace protein • trace carbohydrate

Serve with meat, chicken, tuna or crab sandwiches.

1 egg yolk*

2 tablespoons fresh lime juice

1 tablespoon Dijon mustard

1 tablespoon curry powder

2 teaspoons grated lime zest

freshly ground black pepper, to taste

½ cup pure-pressed extra virgin olive oil

½ cup pure-pressed canola oil

In a blender or food processor, blend egg yolk, lime juice, mustard, curry powder, lime zest and black pepper until smooth. With motor running, gradually drizzle in oils until creamy and thickened. Store covered in refrigerator.

---

*If you are concerned about using raw egg, choose an alternate recipe.

Garlic Caper Mayonnaise

Makes about 1¼ cups • 1 tablespoon: trace protein • trace carbohydrate

Delicious with grilled fish and chicken or as a dip for artichokes or raw vegetables.

1 egg yolk*

2 tablespoons fresh lemon juice

1 minced garlic clove

1 tablespoon drained and rinsed capers

freshly ground black pepper, to taste

dash cayenne pepper

½ cup pure-pressed extra virgin olive oil

½ cup pure-pressed canola oil

2 tablespoons minced fresh parsley

In a blender or food processor, blend egg yolk, lemon juice, garlic, capers and cayenne pepper until smooth. With motor running, gradually add oils until creamy and thickened. Stir in parsley. Taste, and adjust seasonings. Store covered in refrigerator.

———————————

*If you are concerned about using raw egg, choose an alternate recipe.

Pestos

Asian Pesto

Makes about 1 cup • 2 tablespoons: 1 gram protein • 1 gram carbohydrate

Serve with grilled fish or chicken.

1 cup loosely packed fresh mint
  leaves

1 cup loosely packed fresh
  cilantro

1 cup loosely packed fresh basil
  leaves

¼ cup pure-pressed extra virgin
  olive oil

¼ cup chopped raw walnuts

2 tablespoons fresh lime juice

2 minced garlic cloves

freshly ground black pepper,
  to taste

In a blender or food processor, purée all ingredients. Taste, and adjust seasonings. Store covered in refrigerator.

Basil Pesto

Makes about ¾ cup • 2 tablespoons: 6 grams protein • 2 grams carbohydrate

Delicious with grilled fish, chicken or baked potatoes.

2 cups packed fresh basil leaves

2 chopped garlic cloves

3 tablespoons raw pine nuts or raw walnuts

⅓ cup grated Parmesan cheese

⅓ cup pure-pressed extra virgin olive oil

freshly ground black pepper, to taste

dash cayenne pepper

In a blender or food processor, purée all ingredients. Taste, and adjust seasonings. Store covered in refrigerator.

Cilantro Pesto

Makes about 1 cup • 2 tablespoons: 3 grams protein • 2 grams carbohydrate

Serve with grilled fish, chicken or meat, or with cheese quesadillas.

2 bunches cilantro, coarsely chopped with stems removed

2 tablespoons fresh lime juice

½ cup roasted and chopped pumpkin seeds

½ cup grated Parmesan cheese

6 minced garlic cloves

½ cup pure-pressed extra virgin olive oil

freshly ground black pepper, to taste

In a blender or food processor, purée all ingredients. Taste, and adjust seasonings. Store covered in refrigerator.

Sun-Dried Tomato Pesto

Makes about 1 cup • 2 tablespoons: 3 grams protein • 7 grams carbohydrate

Delicious with grilled vegetables, roasted chicken or baked potatoes.

1 cup sun-dried tomatoes in olive oil

2 tablespoons slivered fresh basil, or 1 teaspoon dried basil

¼ cup grated Parmesan cheese

1 minced garlic clove

⅛ teaspoon red-pepper flakes

In a food processor, purée tomatoes with their oil, basil, Parmesan cheese, garlic and red-pepper flakes. Taste, and adjust seasonings. Store covered in refrigerator.

Salsas

Fresh Mexican Salsa

Makes about 2¾ cups • Each ¼ cup serving: trace protein • 2 grams carbohydrate

Serve with grilled vegetables, fish, chicken, meat, cheese quesadillas or enchiladas.

2 cups diced ripe tomatoes

2 minced garlic cloves

2 tablespoons diced red onion

2 tablespoons diced scallions

2 tablespoons minced fresh cilantro

1 small diced fresh jalapeño pepper; or 1 to 2 tablespoons canned diced green chilies, to taste [wear rubber gloves to prepare fresh jalapeño pepper]

2 tablespoons pure-pressed extra virgin olive oil

1 to 2 tablespoons fresh lemon or lime juice, to taste

1 teaspoon dried oregano

freshly ground black pepper, to taste

In a medium bowl, combine all ingredients. Taste, and adjust seasonings. Chill before serving.

Fresh Papaya or Mango Salsa

Makes about 3 cups • Each ¼ cup serving Papaya Salsa: trace protein • 2 grams carbohydrate
Each ¼ cup serving Mango Salsa: trace protein • 6 grams carbohydrate

Serve with grilled chicken, fajitas, fish, shrimp, meat, or with cheese quesadillas or enchiladas.

1 small minced red onion

1 small minced fresh jalapeño pepper; or 1 to 2 tablespoons canned diced green chilies, to taste [wear rubber gloves to prepare fresh jalapeño pepper]

½ cup chopped red bell pepper

2 minced garlic cloves

2 cups diced papaya, or *2 cups diced mango*

1 seeded and chopped ripe tomato*

2 tablespoons chopped fresh cilantro

2 tablespoons chopped scallions

2 tablespoons fresh lime juice

1 tablespoon pure-pressed extra virgin olive oil

freshly ground black pepper, to taste

In a medium bowl, combine all ingredients and mix well. Taste, and adjust seasonings. Refrigerate 1 hour before serving.

---

*To seed tomatoes: Cut tomatoes in half and squeeze gently. Scoop out seeds using a small spoon or your fingers.

Fresh Salsa Verde

Makes about 2 cups • 2 tablespoons: trace protein • trace carbohydrate

Serve with broiled fish, chicken or meat.

½ cup chopped fresh cilantro

½ cup slivered fresh basil

½ cup chopped fresh parsley

½ cup chopped scallions

2 minced garlic cloves

⅓ cup balsamic vinegar

freshly ground black pepper, to taste

1 cup pure-pressed extra virgin olive oil

In a food processor, blend all ingredients except olive oil. With motor running, slowly drizzle in olive oil until well blended. Taste, and adjust seasonings. Store covered in the refrigerator.

Fresh Thai Salsa

Makes about 2¹/₂ cups • Each 2¹/₂ cup serving: trace protein • trace carbohydrate

Serve with roasted or broiled chicken, fish or meat.

2 tablespoons chopped scallions

¹/₃ cup fresh lime juice

2 tablespoons minced fresh cilantro

2 minced garlic cloves

2 tablespoons slivered fresh basil

1 tablespoon minced fresh mint

4 ripe medium tomatoes,
   seeded and diced*

¼ cup diced red onion

2 teaspoons peeled and finely
   minced fresh ginger

1 tablespoon balsamic vinegar

½ cup pure-pressed extra virgin
   olive oil

freshly ground black pepper,
   to taste

In a medium bowl, combine all ingredients. Mix well. Taste, and adjust seasonings. Store covered in refrigerator.

---

*To seed tomatoes: Cut tomatoes in half and squeeze gently. Scoop out seeds using a small spoon or your fingers.

Sauces

Basic Tomato Sauce

Makes about 5 cups • Each ½ cup serving: 1 gram protein • 5 grams carbohydrate

Serve with meatballs and steamed grains.

2 tablespoons pure-pressed extra
    virgin olive oil

1 medium chopped onion

4 minced garlic cloves

28 ounces canned crushed
    tomatoes (reserve liquid)

¼ cup tomato paste

½ cup red wine

1 bay leaf

2 teaspoons dried oregano

¼ teaspoon red-pepper flakes

½ cup slivered fresh basil, or
    2 teaspoons dried basil

¼ cup finely chopped fresh
    parsley

freshly ground black pepper,
    to taste

In a large saucepan, heat oil over medium-high heat. When oil is hot, add onion and garlic and sauté over medium heat until softened, about 5 minutes. Add tomatoes and their liquid, tomato paste, red wine, bay leaf, oregano, red-pepper flakes, basil, parsley and black pepper. Stir well. Bring to a boil. Reduce heat and simmer 30 minutes, stirring occasionally. Taste, and adjust seasonings.

Cilantro Lime Sauce

Makes about 1 cup • 2 tablespoons: trace protein • trace carbohydrate

Serve with fish, chicken, meats or steamed vegetables.

1 stick unsalted butter

½ cup chopped red onion

2 minced garlic cloves

3 tablespoons fresh lime juice

2 teaspoons grated lime zest

dash hot-pepper sauce

2 tablespoons chopped fresh cilantro

freshly ground black pepper, to taste

In a medium nonstick skillet, melt butter over medium-high heat. When butter is hot and bubbly, add onion and garlic and cook until softened, about 5 minutes. Add lime juice, zest, hot-pepper sauce, cilantro and black pepper. Simmer 5 minutes over medium-low heat. Transfer to a blender or food processor and blend until smooth. Taste, and adjust seasonings.

Classic Blender Hollandaise Sauce

Makes about 1 cup • Each ¼ cup serving: 2½ grams protein • trace carbohydrate

Serve with fish, chicken, eggs or steamed vegetables.

3 egg yolks*
2 tablespoons fresh lemon juice
dash cayenne pepper

4 ounces (1 stick) unsalted
butter, melted and bubbling hot

In a blender, combine egg yolks, lemon juice and cayenne pepper, on high for 3 seconds. Remove lid and, with motor running, slowly pour hot butter in a steady stream over eggs. When butter is all poured in, blend an additional 5 seconds. Taste, and adjust seasonings. Serve immediately, or keep sauce warm by placing blender in a bowl of warm water.

---

*If you are concerned about using raw eggs, choose an alternate recipe.

Coconut Curry Sauce

Makes about 1½ cups • Each ¼ cup serving: 2 grams protein • trace carbohydrate

Serve with grilled or baked fish, shrimp, chicken or rice.

1 tablespoon unsalted butter

1½ tablespoons curry powder

2 minced garlic cloves

2 teaspoons peeled and finely
    minced fresh ginger

¼ teaspoon ground cardamom

1 teaspoon mustard seeds

¾ cup all-dairy heavy cream

½ cup coconut milk

1 tablespoon shredded unsweet-
    ened coconut

1 tablespoon minced fresh cilantro

2 teaspoons minced fresh mint

freshly ground black pepper,
    to taste

In a medium saucepan, melt butter over medium-high heat. When butter is hot and bubbly, add curry powder, garlic, ginger, cardamom and mustard seeds. Reduce heat to low and sauté 2 to 3 minutes, until mustard seeds begin to pop.

Add cream, coconut milk, coconut, cilantro, mint and black pepper. Mix well with a wooden spoon. Simmer gently 5 minutes, stirring until thickened and well mixed. Taste, and adjust seasonings.

Cooling Mint Sauce

Makes about 1½ cups • Each ¼ cup serving: 2 grams protein • 2 grams carbohydrate

Serve with Indian main-course curries or lamb dishes.

1 cup whole plain yogurt

½ teaspoon grated lime zest

1 tablespoon finely chopped fresh mint

½ cup peeled, seeded and diced cucumber

In a small bowl, using a fork or wooden spoon, combine yogurt, lime zest, mint and cucumber until well blended. Store covered in refrigerator.

Enchilada Sauce

Makes about 3 cups • Each ½ cup serving: 2 grams protein • 6 grams carbohydrate

Serve with enchiladas, Huevos Rancheros or cheese quesadillas.

2 tablespoons pure-pressed extra virgin olive oil

1 large diced onion

3 minced garlic cloves

1 small minced fresh jalapeño pepper; or 1 to 2 tablespoons canned green chilies, to taste [wear rubber gloves to prepare fresh jalapeño pepper]

2 teaspoons ground cumin

2 teaspoons dried oregano

2 teaspoons chili powder

freshly ground black pepper, to taste

28 ounces canned tomatoes, puréed (reserve liquid)

1 to 2 tablespoons fresh lime juice, to taste

1 tablespoon minced fresh cilantro

In a large nonstick saucepan, heat oil over medium-high heat. When oil is hot, add onion, garlic, jalapeño pepper, cumin, oregano, chili powder and black pepper. Sauté until onion is softened, about 5 minutes. Add tomatoes and their liquid, mix well and bring to a boil. Reduce heat to low, and simmer uncovered 15 to 20 minutes. Add lime juice and minced cilantro. Taste, and adjust seasonings.

Herbed Caper Butter

Makes about ½ cup • 1 tablespoon: trace protein • trace carbohydrate

Serve with fish, chicken, steamed vegetables or baked potatoes.

4 tablespoons unsalted butter

1 tablespoon drained and rinsed
capers

1 tablespoon fresh lemon juice

1 teaspoon dried oregano

freshly ground black pepper,
to taste

In a small saucepan, melt butter over low heat. When butter is melted, add remaining ingredients. Heat through. Taste, and adjust seasonings. Serve warm.

Horseradish Sauce

Makes about 1 cup • 2 tablespoons serving: 1 gram protein • 1 gram carbohydrate

Excellent with meat or poached fish.

2 tablespoons horseradish

¾ cup whole sour cream

1 tablespoon Dijon mustard

½ teaspoon white vinegar

freshly ground black pepper,
to taste

In a medium bowl, using a fork, combine all ingredients and mix well. Taste, and adjust seasonings. Refrigerate before serving.

Mustard Sauce

Makes about 1½ cups • Each ¼ cup serving: 1 gram protein • trace carbohydrate

Delicious with grilled fish, chicken and meats.

2 egg yolks*	*1 minced garlic clove*
2 teaspoons red wine vinegar	*3 tablespoons Dijon mustard*
dash white pepper	*1 cup pure-pressed canola oil*
1 tablespoon fresh lemon juice	

In a blender or food processor, blend all ingredients except oil. With motor running, drizzle in oil until sauce is smooth. Taste, and adjust seasonings. Store covered in refrigerator.

---

*If you are concerned about using raw eggs, choose an alternate recipe.

Quick Blender Béarnaise Sauce

Makes about 1½ cups • Each ¼ cup serving: 2 grams protein • trace carbohydrate

Delicious with fish, chicken, omelets and meat.

2 tablespoons white wine	*3 egg yolks**
1 tablespoon tarragon vinegar	*2 tablespoons fresh lemon juice*
1 tablespoon chopped fresh	*dash cayenne pepper*
tarragon	*½ cup melted, bubbly hot*
1 tablespoon chopped shallots	*unsalted butter*
¼ teaspoon black pepper	

In a small saucepan, combine wine, vinegar, tarragon, shallots and pepper. Bring to a boil and reduce by half.

In a blender, combine egg yolks with lemon juice and cayenne pepper, on high. With motor running, gradually drizzle in hot melted butter. Add herb/wine mixture and blend on high until creamy and thickened. Taste and adjust seasonings.

---

*If you are concerned about using raw eggs, choose an alternate recipe.

Shitake Mushroom Gravy

Makes about 2¼ cups • Each 2 tablespoon serving: trace protein • trace carbohydrate

1 ounce dried shitake mushrooms

2 tablespoons unsalted butter

1 medium chopped onion

1 minced garlic clove

2 tablespoons dry sherry

1 teaspoon paprika

1 tablespoon low-sodium tamari soy sauce

4 tablespoons butter

3 tablespoons flour

2 cups reserved shitake mushroom soaking liquid or vegetable stock (see recipe, page 115), heated

2 tablespoons chopped fresh parsley

freshly ground black pepper, to taste

Cover shitake mushrooms with 3 cups hot water and let stand for about 20 minutes. Remove from water, strain liquid and set aside. Cut coarse stem end off of mushrooms and discard. Slice mushroom caps into ¼ inch strips.

In a large skillet, melt 2 tablespoons butter over medium-high heat. When butter is hot and bubbly, add onions, garlic and mushrooms. Sauté 8 minutes, stirring frequently.

Add sherry, paprika and soy sauce and cook 1 minute before transferring mushroom mixture to a bowl.

Melt 4 tablespoons butter in pan over medium-high heat. When butter is hot and bubbly, add flour and whisk, stirring and cooking for 5 minutes.

Meanwhile, heat reserved mushroom liquid or stock to almost boiling. Slowly add hot mushroom liquid or stock to butter and flour mixture. Cook until thickened, stirring frequently, about 5 minutes.

Stir in sautéed mushroom mixture, parsley and black pepper. Taste, and adjust seasonings. Serve as is or blend in food processor or blender until smooth.

Spicy Cocktail Sauce

Makes about 1¼ cups • Each ⅓ cup serving: trace protein • 1 gram carbohydrate

Serve with seafood.

⅔ cup mayonnaise (made from
  pure-pressed oil)

⅓ cup whole sour cream

1 teaspoon grated lime zest

1 tablespoon fresh lime juice

1 tablespoon chopped fresh
  cilantro or parsley

2 to 3 tablespoons chili sauce,
  to taste

freshly ground black pepper,
  to taste

In a small bowl, using a fork, mix all ingredients until well blended. Taste, and adjust seasonings.

Spicy Peanut Sauce

Makes about 1¼ cups • Each ¼ cup serving: 4 grams protein • 4 grams carbohydrate

Serve with grilled meat, chicken, tofu or steamed brown rice.

5 chopped garlic cloves

2 tablespoons peeled and finely
  minced fresh ginger

½ cup chopped fresh cilantro

2 tablespoons pure-pressed
  sesame oil

1 tablespoon hot chili oil

½ cup organic peanut butter
  (no honey or sugar added)

¼ cup low-sodium tamari soy
  sauce

2 tablespoons fresh lime juice

1 tablespoon rice wine vinegar

dash cayenne pepper

hot water, if needed, to thin

In a food processor, blend garlic, ginger and cilantro. Add oils, peanut butter, soy sauce, lime juice, vinegar and cayenne pepper and blend until smooth and creamy, scraping down sides of bowl. Add hot water for a thinner consistency. Taste, and adjust seasonings, adding more soy sauce or lime juice, if desired.

Tartar Sauce

Makes about 1¼ cups • 2 tablespoons serving: trace protein • trace carbohydrate

Serve with seafood.

1 cup mayonnaise (made from
   pure-pressed oil)

1 teaspoon Dijon mustard

1 tablespoon unsweetened pickle
   relish

1 tablespoon drained and rinsed
   capers

1 tablespoon minced scallions

1 tablespoon minced fresh parsley

2 tablespoons fresh lemon juice

freshly ground black pepper,
   to taste

In a medium bowl, combine all ingredients, mixing well with a fork. Taste, and adjust seasonings. Refrigerate before serving.

Index

About the Authors

Diana Schwarzbein, M.D., graduated from the University of Southern California (USC) Medical School and completed her residency in internal medicine and a fellowship in endocrinology at Los Angeles County USC Medical Center. She founded The Endrocrinology Institute of Santa Barbara in 1993. She sub-specializes in metabolism, diabetes, osteoporosis, menopause and thyroid conditions, subjects she lectures on frequently. She lives with her husband in Santa Barbara, California.

Nancy Deville is a writer of fiction and nonfiction with a talent for making science easy to read and understand. She recently completed a novel and screenplay about trafficking in women. She is currently at work on a second novel and a nonfiction book. She is a contributing writer on *Legacy: Secrets of Family Business Dynasties,* to be published by St. Martins Press. She lives with her husband in Santa Barbara, California.

Evelyn Jacob Jaffe combines her love of cooking with her artistic talents. She is the former co-owner of the New York Bagel Factory of Santa Barbara and the founder and former director of Project Food Chain, a program that provides meals for people with AIDS and other life-challenging illnesses. She currently works as a private executive chef and caterer, as well as developing recipes for gourmet food companies. She lives with her husband and two sons in Carpinteria, California.

Diana Schwarzbein, M.D., Nancy Deville and Evelyn Jacob Jaffe are also the authors of *The Schwarzbein Principle Vegetarian Cookbook.*

The Schwarzbein Principle
The Latest Evolution in Health and Fitness

Adopt this Five-Step Nutrition and Lifestyle Program
You deserve it!

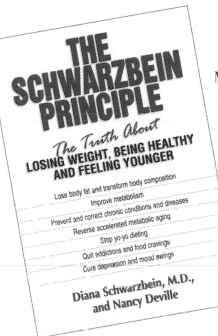

Maximize your metabolism and
achieve lasting weight loss with
The Schwarzbein Principle.
Through real-life stories, this
book reveals how excess
weight, "Accelerated aging"
and degenerative disease
can be controlled and
reversed.

Code #6803 • $12.95

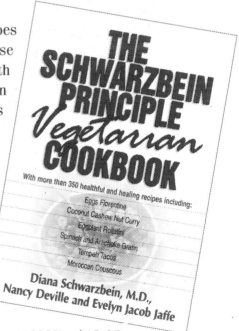